Back to Nursing with Confidence

The complete guide for a nurse returning to the profession following a substantial break, with up-to-date and practical information about the world of modern nursing.

A Letter to the NURSING MIRROR, 14 August 1985

NEVER TOO LATE

Forty-two years of age, children old enough to look after themselves. What should I do with myself? Go back to nursing, everyone said. I had left 16 years previously, would it have changed very much?

My chance came. A friend asked me if I would be interested in a part-time staff nurse's post on night duty at a private nursing home. There I learned some of the new techniques and drugs. I realised there had been changes and wondered if I would be able to cope in a big hospital. In the meantime I put my name down for a part-time post at a women's hospital.

Six months later, a post became vacant. I was given a date for an interview. Would I be able to give the right answers? Would the fact that I was as yet unfamiliar with some of the modern techniques be a disadvantage?

Day of the interview dawned and I went off, stomach full of butterflies. I was met by the nursing officer who showed me to her office where my future ward sister was waiting. They both soon made me feel at ease. The interview seemed to go without a hitch, though the ward sister did have some reservations as to whether I would be able to cope with nurses young enough to be my daughters giving me orders. But she was willing to give me a trial.

First day on the ward feeling just like a first year. I need not have worried, everyone made me feel part of the team. The young nurses have never treated me as anything other than one of them.

Things had changed. Everything came made up in packs. I thought I would never learn all the new drugs, operations and, most of all, the nursing process, though basic nursing never changes and the patient still relies on you as a nurse.

First time in charge—would I do something silly? But I need not have worried. I had a good team of nurses with me, and they helped me through. Six months soon went by and I found everything fitting into place and myself fitting into the ward.

It is now two years since I made that step back to nursing. My advice to ex-nurses: 'Take the bull by the horns and come back.' You may be out of touch but your past experience and your knowledge of life outside nursing is the greatest gift you can pass on to the young nurses training now.

A. Murphy,
Birmingham.

Back to Nursing with Confidence

Irene Heywood Jones
SRN RMN ONC DipN RNT

Heinemann Nursing
London

First published 1986
by William Heinemann Medical Books
23 Bedford Square
London WC1B 3HH

ISBN 0–433–14710–5

Photoset and printed in Great Britain by
Redwood Burn Limited, Trowbridge, Wiltshire

Contents

Preface

Voluntary self-help groups. Community health council. Health service commissioner. Preventive health care. Health education. The patient's day.

For the purposes of this book, to make easy reading, nurses are in the female gender and patients are in the male gender.

Journalism is not about *what* you know but about *who* you know and *where* to find the necessary information. I am indebted to the countless numbers of people who were so helpful in providing the facts, enabling me to compile this book, which I hope will be of benefit to the readers.

A thanks as well to Barbara Christopher SRN, also a returned nurse, for her perceptive sketches.

Preface

At the outset of their nursing career, most young girls appreciate the value of pursuing a training that will stand them in good stead for the future. They also realise, with sound justification, that should they ever wish to take a break in service to raise a family, nursing is a job to which they could return and could choose from a wide range of opportunities that require the basic nursing qualification.

It is not always easy or economically viable to make alternative arrangements to allow a young mother to continue her career while bringing up a family. Many women manage some part-time nursing, whereas others make a conscious choice to be full-time mothers, until the children are well established at school.

Busily occupied with two or three children, it is easy to become steeped in domestic responsibilities, as your world revolves around the needs of the family and it is difficult to remember those carefree student days, when meals were served to you! Although the career part of you recedes into the distance temporarily, the core of your knowledge and that valuable experience remains, and is indeed built upon, by maturity.

When the little ones grow and seek independence, they leave their mother the freedom to regain herself, to pick up the threads of her professional life, with some 20 to 30 potential working years stretching ahead.

The thought of returning to work feels exciting. The enjoyment of adult company, the buzz of a busy environment, learning anew, participating in progressive techniques, being needed, feeling good about helping patients and their relatives. You remember how much you used to enjoy the job, the thrill of belonging to a functioning team, the involvement, the responsibility and the personal pride in a satisfactory day—even the anxieties of a not so satisfactory day. And some extra money would be very useful too.

Despite the attraction of the emotional and financial rewards, doubts begin to creep in as to whether you could cope with the role and responsibility of a trained nurse. After an absence of 5, 7, 10 or maybe 15 years with your boundaries limited to the home, you wonder what life is really like back in the big world of work. You are apprehensive that the nursing profession may have changed beyond recognition, that things are not done now as you were taught, that drugs are different and techniques have altered. Does the nursing today resemble what you learnt? What do you have to offer? What could your contribution be to contemporary patient care? Could you master the changes in the time warp? Dare you plan any further?

Read on.

1

Mothers and Nursing— Why Work?

My family and friends were amazed at the change in me when I returned to work—and, frankly, so was I. After so long at home, I'd lost all my confidence and was terrified silly about going back into hospital work but I knew I had to. At 37, I had a lifetime ahead of me and wasn't going to idle it away. I believed that I did have a lot to offer and, with the assurance that I had had a good basic training in my background, I nervously hurtled in and soon found my feet.

I became a different person once I took on outside responsibility, more lively, more sure of myself, interesting and interested in other things. That was funny really. Even though I was busy at the hospital and coping with the home, because I was stimulated and happy I found renewed energy to pursue extra activities with the new friends I had made.

It was as if someone had plugged me back into the real world; I had rejoined the human race and found myself again. I didn't have time to dwell on aches or pains, to wallow in depression or boredom, as I had been inclined to do before. I was too occupied in many directions and never looked back after taking that initial step to return to work.

Violet, mother of three children, whose ages span over a 10-year period, returned to work as a staff nurse in an outpatient department, after 14 years out of nursing. She had attended nurse refresher courses occasionally during this absence.

I love my work, I love my children, but there is no way that I could bear to be confined to the home, I'd go scatty without some intellectual stimulation! It is a considerable outlay for a day nanny, but worth every penny to allow me to pursue my career while they are well cared for. I am so much happier, the children adore the girl and we lead a full life as a family.

Karen has two preschool children, works full-time as a nurse tutor, during which time she studied for a degree with some assisted leave extended to tutorial staff. With the backup of a supportive husband and an excellent childcare arrangement, she is planning to take maternity leave to have a third child.

After my second daughter was born and I'd been at home for three years, I was desperate to get out of the house and back to a working environment, even if only for brief periods. I was sick to the back teeth of talking about babies and the price of pork chops. I really missed the stimulation and challenge of nursing, and especially missed the contact with colleagues with whom I could 'talk shop'.

And I was heartily fed up with having no money of my own. I resented needing to ask my husband every time that I wanted my hair done or a pair of tights, after I had been used to my own income.

I wanted to be more than a housewife and mother and was anxious to regain an identity of my own. I felt I was in a void, just vegetating at home. When I found myself sitting watching TV in the afternoon, I had to believe there was more to life than that!

Mary worked through a nurse bank scheme whenever her husband's shift allowed him to babysit. She later joined the staff and subsequently became night sister on the intensive therapy unit.

I was terrified at the thought of returning to work after a 15-year break. I felt *so* out of touch, yet the need for some extra cash and a longing to return to midwifery spurred me on.

A mother of four from Scotland who returned to midwifery.

When I was pregnant, I resigned from my work, but returned within a year, having second thoughts about full-time mothering.

A clinical teacher with access to a hospital crèche is about to take maternity leave for the forthcoming birth of her second baby.

When my husband was suddenly made redundant, we were jolly thankful that I had a training to fall back on.

Susan had no choice but to return to full-time nursing after a six-year absence.

These are the testimonies of some nurses who decided to combine work with motherhood in some way, at some time in their lives. Their statements are not for scrutiny, criticism or public debate. They are the candid gut reactions surrounding the decision taken by each woman, in the light of her own needs and practical considerations for her family. In our contemporary society, there is no right way, no wrong way—only personal choice that is correct for each individual family (see Figure 1.1).

Should a woman decide *not* to work, then that is right for her.

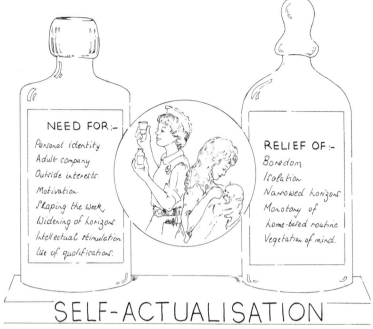

NEED FOR:-

Personal identity.
Adult company.
Outside interests.
Motivation.
Shaping the week.
Widening of horizons.
Intellectual stimulation.
Use of qualifications.

RELIEF OF:-

Boredom.
Isolation.
Narrowed horizons.
Monotony of
home-based routine.
Vegetation of mind.

SELF-ACTUALISATION

Fig. 1.1

Giving a woman the 'opportunity', by legislation or provision of childcare options, facilitates her ability to work, if she so chooses—but in no way makes it compulsory!

Similarly, in some instances women do not have a reasonable choice either way should adverse circumstances dictate their lifestyle, for instance, in cases of the single, deserted, divorced or widowed mother, or one whose husband is out of work.

Some women would not opt to work before their children were of reasonable age and level of independence. In no way would they be prepared to assume the dual role, possibly feeling that this would either compromise their responsibility to their children or their patients. Neither do they feel able to see their way around the necessarily intricate organisation of their life which can at times resemble a juggling act!

Nothing would induce me to find work of any sort, I have quite enough to do at home. I cannot begin to imagine how these women manage; I like a simple, orderly existence and am keen to avoid hassle, not add to it.

This was from a mother who has decided not to return to nursing, even though she frequently finds she is helping out friends who have got a job and a family.

Conversely, some women are determined to continue with their chosen career, as well as having children, and make the necessary arrangements to permit this.

Between these two extremes are a variety of ways to mix and match work and family life, at some stage, whether it be sooner or later. It is only natural for a trained nurse to look to her profession, to see what she has to offer it—and what it has to offer her.

For example, many mothers feel it is their prime duty to dedicate themselves to stay at home with preschool children, although they are happy to seek suitable employment that will fit in with the needs of the family. A nurse with a shift-working husband finds she can fit in some work via an agency or a nurse bank. Or the odd night shift can seem an attractive proposition when the husband can babysit. Some women, who during an exhausting pregnancy relished the thought of a break from work to enjoy motherhood, may become disillusioned with the new lifestyle and wish to seek some outside interest.

Somewhere along the way, you will sense what is right for you and your family, what you need and can personally manage—then you will seek to achieve it.

For every woman rushing to get her baby to the childminder before a busy day on the ward, there is another mother clearing up the toyroom and running the toddler club. For every working woman employing a minder or a nanny, there is a career mother busily caring for someone else's child. Each must respect the other's choice as right for that particular woman.

For every joyful full-time mother, there is her counterpart who is suffocating and frustrated at being all day in the house with tiny children.

Why return to work?

There are many reasons why women want to work, each of differing importance for different individuals but they fall into three major areas of need:

- self-actualisation

- money
- career development

Self-actualisation

Looking after young children all day has some highs, some lows, and an awful lot of mediocre tedium in between. Children require constant supervision and stimulation of activities at their level of development. The adult in total charge must get down to the child's level of communication and adapt to the child's pace.

No one can deny the crucial needs of the growing child, but such an existence can have a demoralising effect on the person in full-time charge. The adult mind is not stretched or challenged, so it stagnates more easily and one forgets precisely how to exercise it on adult topics.

A nurse who has been used to a busy, demanding, responsible life, using her brain and making important decisions, can find full-time motherhood a pretty stultifying experience. Worse still is that after several years of being dormant, she may doubt her ability ever to get back to her former competence, enthusiasm, quickwittedness, efficiency and communication on professional matters.

In short, being away from the work scene for any length of time reduces confidence considerably, as well as making one take a sharp look at one's own identity and value. The same can happen to those who retire or are made redundant, when they have lost the crutch of work and are forced to reassess and replan their lives.

Each presents a case of profound culture shock.

With our modern society of the mobile nuclear family—one mother, one father, 2.3 children—mothers have lost support from the extended family and are forced to build a new circle of contacts. Granny, sister, auntie may no longer live close by, to lend a helping hand to a new mother and give her occasional relief from the baby. In a world of pushbutton automated housework, the mother and child relationship becomes unnaturally claustrophobic, in contrast to the days when they both shared in feeding the chickens or hanging out the washing.

New mothers can suffer a tremendous sense of isolation, especially if they have previously been to work and not developed friends or acquaintances in the locality. One big benefit of antenatal classes, infant clinics and the National Childbirth Trust is to provide essential contacts for mothers within their own neighbourhood.

It is within the nature of things that mothers are flung together with those similarly placed and the conversation inevitably centres on the development of the children, as the obvious focal point of contact. Toddlers need other toddlers to play with, so a mother must foster relationships with people who, like herself, have suitable toys, have packed away their china ornaments and don't object to orange juice being spilt on the carpet!

All of this enforces a very restricted perspective on life and can become very tiresome on a daily basis.

The main complaint from mothers with young children is a severe narrowing of horizons. Outings with children are limited—witness a toddler tantrum in a department store! Outings without children usually require expensive or elaborate arrangements.

With the best will in the world, trying to get involved in a meaningful conversation on a general topic is extremely difficult when toddlers interrupt at frequent intervals. It is hardly surprising that women may just give up in frustration, feel beaten into submission, and allow their minds to fix in neutral for a few years.

It is the precise aim of an organisation such as the National Housewives Register to try to counteract this regressive step, by encouraging involvement in matters of general interest. It brings housewives together for stimulating talks and discussions on a wide variety of topics, provided that they have nothing to do with the home or children. It is a useful, invigorating mental and social experience away from the house, as are evening or day classes, some of which do have a crèche.

In our modern society, housekeeping and motherhood as a chosen avenue of lifestyle is given low social prestige, which is a shame and totally unfair to those women who enjoy the role and do it well. A woman becomes relegated to being 'someone's wife' and 'someone's mother', thereby losing her own identity and with it, very often, her self-esteem.

A mother's day, indeed a mother's week, has little structure to it. The chores roll along in one continuum, as even the child's feeding and sleeping takes a while to settle into a pattern. There is no off-duty time at 4.30 pm, the responsibility continues through the day and the night, there are no paid holidays from motherhood and no sick leave either. You only fully realise *this* when you are feeling deathly with flu, but still have two lively infants bouncing around and needing your attention! Work gives some shape to the day and something to look forward to, which will ring the changes.

Increasingly disillusioned with the reality of constant mothering, some women feel that the best option all round is to arrange for someone to care for the children, get out of the house, seek some stimulation and breathe a different atmosphere. They feel the urge to talk about things they understand and enjoy and want to utilise their skills in a working environment that they find familiar and comfortable.

Alternatively, the mother who had settled happily to home life with small children, may have *her* personal crisis at a later stage. When the children are confidently off to school, mother may find the day hangs heavily around her after the housework has been speedily despatched. It is not unknown for a new baby to be born to fill the gap left by the departure of the youngest child to school!

So a woman may want to work for the personal satisfaction that she alone can derive from being back in the work situation— to stretch her mind, to enjoy the responsibility of a worthwhile contribution to society, to learn new things and to teach others, to have adult contact and adult interests. Nursing may be tiring but it is never boring.

It is a delight to relate to other staff and patients, to feel part of a constructive team, and the week has some reference points. Nurses adore getting together to 'talk shop', just as members of other professions enjoy meeting up with their colleagues.

In addition, there may be the social spinoffs from being back at work, such as making new friends, joining in activities arranged by groups of staff and generally adding an extra dimension to your life.

So much has been said about 'fulfilment' that it has become a rather hackneyed word. Spinsters used to be unfulfilled because they did not have children. Mothers may now be unfulfilled because they have lost their career.

The dictionary defines it 'to develop and realise the potential of...'. Only you know what is your potential, within the family and work situations, and how you intend to develop it. Fulfilment is achievement of different aims at different levels for different people—there is no accepted norm to emulate.

For me, going to work is like having a day off. Being able to be myself and indulge in my own interest for two days allows me to enjoy the remainder of the week. It has also been very valuable that I have been able to maintain useful contact with professional developments.

These are words from a part-time tutor with two preschool children cared for by a childminder.

Money

Everybody can make use of some extra money, although nursing has never been a particularly highly paid job. Financial gain may be a lesser or greater incentive for mothers to seek employment. In a survey of American working mothers, three-quarters admitted they would choose to continue working, even if their financial situation were to improve dramatically.

Money might be essential to a lone mother or a wife whose husband is unemployed but care must be taken that any income does not jeopardise social security benefits or pension, in the case of a widow.

For wives who have always had to share their husband's income, it is tremendously satisfying to have some degree of financial independence.

The nurse returning to work needs to reckon the earnings that she will receive in relation to her outgoings and this may influence the pattern of work that she decides to undertake. She will need to take account of any expenses incurred with respect to childcare, travel and meals, tax and insurance.

Nurses do not need to purchase or launder expensive work clothes as uniforms are part of the job; however, agency nurses are expected to provide their own uniform, either privately or through the agency.

Reasonably priced meals can be bought in the hospital cafeteria—a cooked meal is often seen as a luxury for the woman who does not have to cook it.

All working nurses will have national insurance contributions deducted pro rata to their salary. Nurses appointed to the staff are eligible for sick and holiday pay and perhaps maternity benefit and leave after a qualifying period. Bank nurses and agency nurses do not get any paid holiday leave or sick pay.

Paid contributions for superannuation will vary depending upon the hours worked. If working under half the full-time hours (at present it is half of 37½ = 18¾ hours per week) no nurse can be included in the superannuation scheme. But if she works over the half-time hours and up to the full-time hours, she may choose to pay into the scheme, which also commits the employing authority to a similar contribution. Once the nurse is in full-time employment, she has no choice and contribution is deducted at source, added to the contribution of the employer on her behalf. Some nurses deliberately keep their hours just below the full-time amount (even to 37 hours), so as to avoid that deduction from their salary.

However, it is worth looking carefully at the benefits of the superannuation scheme, which provides a pension, especially if you have many more years ahead to work before retiring age.

Everybody is permitted to earn a certain tax-free amount annually, known as the single person's allowance. Beyond that level, all income is subject to tax at a calculated percentage. For a married woman, her income is added to her husband's income for this calculation, unless she opts for separate taxation.

A nurse contemplating work needs to assess whether it will be worth her while financially to work hours which incur childcare expenses, especially if this has to be deducted from salary that has already been taxed.

She may find it suits her better to be employed through an agency or a bank, so she can pick her hours, thereby choosing to work more during term time and less during school holidays. A nurse who is employed on the staff must take note of these occasional expenses if she is unable to juggle with her hours.

A nurse may prefer to work one long night shift which would equate with the pay for several short day shifts and incur less overall expense for travel.

Working unsocial hours can indeed push up the level of basic pay considerably, and an increased rate of pay is as follows.

- night work, that is evenings
  after 8 pm   = time + a third
- all day Saturday   = time + a third
- all day Sunday   = time + two-thirds
- bank holidays   = time + two-thirds + a day
                                   off in lieu

Certain less desirable specialties carry an extra allowance or 'lead'; this applies to geriatrics, the chronic sick, the younger disabled and psychiatric nursing, which has an additional payment for those working in secure units or special hospitals.

When a nurse returns to her career after a break in service, her previous experience will be credited when estimating her pay scale. For example, if she left six years ago, having reached fourth year staff nurse grade, then she will recommence employment at fourth year staff nurse level. It may take some time for the finance department to verify these periods of experience with former employees, which is necessary before the correct level of payment can be assigned to the new nurse.

The finance department will always be pleased to help with any queries over matters of pay, and they will refer to the manual issued by the Nursing and Midwifery Staffs Negotiating Council (formerly Whitley Council), where all the regulations are clearly detailed.

A back-to-nursing course is likely to include a session for discussion on matters of pay and employment with the finance officer, which can be useful for nurses who have yet to make a final decision about their future employment.

Career development

Heated debate surrounds the issue of women's capability and suitability to hold senior positions, controlling staff and budget, doing battle with other bosses and the unions.

Some would argue that women do not possess the necessary characteristics for the tough life of top level management: drive, aggression, tenacity, ruthlessness, stamina. These qualities are generally ascribed to men, whose other asset is the support of a wife in the background to sustain the flow of his creature comforts. No, women have the psychological makeup comprising tenderness, care, understanding, that equips them ideally for the rearing of children. That's where they should stay and, anyway, someone has got to do it!

This line of thought resolves with the firm idea that women should not attempt to mix work—well not *serious* work—with raising a family. There is already sufficient competition from the single women who have dug their heels in to climb the ladder of success, without having the added complication of women with heavy domestic responsibilities.

Whatever the truth may be, attitudes die hard and, despite helpful laws about the employment of women, it is the basic attitude that prejudices their chances.

There is, in fact, plenty of evidence to suggest that everybody is subjected to social conditioning and will respond largely to what is expected of them.

A wonderfully graphic experiment shows how sexual stereotyping begins from early conditioning, to become ingrained in the mores of tradition.

A baby is dressed in a pink, frilly dress, called 'Angela' and handed to the adult subject. The subject talks of the baby being 'fine, delicate, precious, beautiful', while gently cooing and lulling, and choosing for 'Angela' a smiling, soft doll.

When the same baby is dressed in a blue romper suit, called 'Tom' and handed to the same adult, there is a dramatic alteration in the subject's behaviour. This 'boy' is a 'toughy, a real lad, full of life, strong', as he is jiggled and bounced, chuckled and romped into animation, with the help of a noisy rattle chosen from a selection of toys.

Yet people have different talents, different attributes that they should be allowed to develop, without the rigid preconceived sexual stereotyping. A lot of very useful gifts will be lost if that rigid rule is applied and people may be pigeonholed into a lifestyle which makes them profoundly unhappy. Not *all* men will be suitable for top managerial jobs, just as not *all* women will be unsuitable for those posts. Some men would welcome spending more time at home, just as some women would enjoy a break from it occasionally.

Growing children are now given plenty of opportunity to try their hand at a variety of skills across the sexual barrier. Girls are encouraged to study physics and science and to join in the woodwork classes, while their male peers attend classes in cookery and childcare. Both participate in computer studies.

There is a greater overlap of roles, and consequently girls now have higher expectations of their achievement potential. A job is not seen as 'something to do until Mr Right comes along on bended knee with a marriage proposal'. A career is something within their grasp—and grasp it they will.

Marriage no longer signifies the automatic end to the working life of a woman—indeed, quite the opposite, when her wages make a necessary contribution to the mortgage commitment and household expenses. The arrival of children may be the time when a woman decides to leave work or chooses to take maternity leave which entitles her to job security.

It is unlawful to dismiss an employee on the grounds of pregnancy. If a woman has been with the same employer for the previous two years, she is entitled to paid leave and up to 29 weeks away from work after the confinement. Her job *must* be kept open and, in the health service, she can request to return on a part-time basis at the same grade, although it may involve a change in area of work.

Now fertility can be controlled and a conscious decision made when to interrupt work to have children, two fairly distinct career patterns for women tend to emerge.

(1) The woman who opts to defer her career will elect for marriage and children earlier, rather than later, perhaps in her early to mid-20s. She is then freed from critical mothering responsibilities by the time she takes up her career again towards her 40s. This may appeal to the nurse who, having secured a useful, basic qualification, feels confident to take a break, as she can resume her career at a later stage. She will miss out on training and promotion prospects during this absence but can realistically catch up, provided that she is adequately updated.

This younger mother, who will probably be at a modest level in the profession—on an equally modest salary—may find it uneconomical to continue working if she has to pay for childcare. Although nursery and childminder fees are reasonable for one child, they increase with subsequent children and may make full-time work hardly worth the bother, if financial gain is the main criterion.

Many of these women recognise that their career has to be 'kept on ice' during the childrearing years. They accept this as a small sacrifice for the sake of having a family and are happy to pay the price of forfeiting their own career advancement. Those who manage any part-time nursing along the way do so provided that it does not incur too much expense and will benefit their career by 'keeping a foot in the door'. Almost without realising, they will absorb the gradual changes occurring within the profession, keep up with new terminology, absorb information through the nursing magazines, maintain their confidence and, possibly, be included on courses. These women, naturally, will find it less of a jolt when they do decide to launch their career full-time in a positive direction.

(2) The other career pattern, which is on the increase especially among professional women, is to defer motherhood. Having become established in a profession and climbing the career ladder, a woman may be reluctant to give up a job which is immensely satisfying and carries an enhanced salary. Yet, as she approaches her mid to late 30s, the woman realises that her child-bearing days are limited and she must act now, or give up the idea of having children at all. So the trend is for couples to delay the start of a family, and the wife enters the medical jargon as an 'elderly primipara'. Unmarried women can also suffer the pangs for last-minute babies and may choose to have a child, which they can support alone, confidently, with a good job behind them.

Now the older mother has much more to lose—what she has attained and wishes to retain of status in her profession, as well as the substantial financial reward. As she earns considerably more, she can afford to employ a nanny or live-in help for full-time sub-stitute mothering. With this arrangement, any subsequent child-ren become absorbed into the initial salary of the nanny, so a larger family does not produce diminishing returns.

About three-quarters of all nurses do have a substantial break in service at some time during their lives and this will affect their professional career.

In nursing, any career enhancement upwards in the profession is geared almost exclusively to full-time staff, who tend to have a record of continuity of service and are flexible to move jobs and take on extended duties related to their role.

Courses of a general educational nature, not connected with promotion, are given to nurses in the lower grades but may still be reserved for full-time staff. It is an enlightened authority that will invest time and money in the career development of its part-time or occasional staff, rather than viewing them as a piece-working pair of hands.

In nursing the majority of top jobs are held by single people, while the majority of married people fill those at staff nurse level, and we can safely assume that many of those will be part-timers. As Table 1.1 shows, in one survey, fully 74.8% of nurse managers were single people, while 78.3% of staff nurses and midwives were married people.

Table 1.1   Designation of nurses by post and marital status

	Single No.	Single %	Married No.	Married %
Administrators	92	74.8	26	21.1
Sisters/teachers	55	51.9	46	43.4
Staff nurses/midwives	23	19.3	93	78.4
Health visitors	28	71.8	11	28.2

Note: Totals do not add up to 100% because other categories (eg divorced) have been omitted
Taken from Hockey L. (1976), *Women in Nursing*, with kind permission of Hodder & Stoughton.

The loss of women from nursing and their relegation to lower grades when working part-time has also contributed to the sharp increase in men securing the top jobs in nursing administration and teaching. Men are very much less likely to work part-time than are women. Table 1.2, based on some Scottish statistics, illustrates this. For example, while 17 704 female RGNs were found to work part-time, only 37 male RGNs did.

So there are clear career advantages of not taking a break from service, but there are logistic difficulties of many types when a woman is constrained by children and the demands of her hus-

Table 1.2   A breakdown of figures on male and female nurses working full-time and part-time

		Whole-time	Part-time
General	Male	1175	37
	Female	21166	17704
Mental health	Male	2620	95
	Female	4971	2618
Mental deficiency	Male	673	16
	Female	1684	680
Maternity	Male	4	—
	Female	3075	2161
Community	Male	104	1
	Female	4005	1383

From SHHD (1978). *Scottish Health Statistics*. Edinburgh: HMSO.

band's job. They have compromises to make that do not affect the lives of single women or married men within the profession.

In essence, career and motherhood are two conflicting forces, but women are increasingly wanting to include both in their lives. It does require extremely careful planning, to ensure that it works happily for the mother, the employer and the child. Many employers fear that working mothers will be unreliable and have divided loyalties, so the woman must try extra hard not to let the two roles interfere with one another unreasonably. A nurse who wishes to pursue her career has to do it wholeheartedly but, in any of the possible circumstances, the final plaintive cry will be: 'What about the children?'. . . .

Childcare options

It takes a generation or so for attitudes to changes in society to reach the man (or woman) in the street. Despite a lot of current idealist talk about the blurring of roles, it is less likely to apply to returning nurses, whose families, like the majority, are still held in the fairly traditional family pattern—father has a steady job and is the breadwinner, while mother has the ultimate responsibility of the children and running the home. Although her financial contribution is welcome to the household, if she wants to work it is generally down to her to make arrangements for childcare and domestic help.

There *are* executive females with nannies and incredibly accommodating husbands, even a new species known as the 'house husband', but these ladies call the tune because they are the essential high earner of the household. If she is called to a foreign conference, it is the man who takes the helm at home.

This situation is unlikely to occur where the wife is a nurse, merely because nursing is not a highly paid occupation. On the whole, any work that a woman can fit in while the children are young is a perk for her in terms of personal satisfaction and 'pin' money. What it must not do is to pose serious competition or threaten disruption to the work of the breadwinning husband, whose job must come first.

If you think you have an equal marriage/job arrangement, ask yourself a few questions. Who takes time from work when measles manifests itself in a child at 7 am? Who arranges to be free to attend sports day and the Christmas concert? Whose job dictates the date of the annual holiday? Who prepares the lunchboxes, the harvest offering and ensures there are clean socks and knickers for all?

In Britain, half of all mothers return to some paid work before their children go to school and there are very few women who are not working by the time their children have reached their teens.

Nursery and crèche facilities for British children are notoriously sparse, compared with many continental countries for whom it is an automatic state provision. Yet a government faced with a tight budget, as well as a tremendous unemployment problem, is hardly likely to give high priority to providing nurseries to enable mothers to work and be free to compete for the jobs that are available.

Private childcare arrangements have to be made, which are of variable expense, make an additional dent in the take-home pay of any working mother, and can prove counterproductive to the very low-paid worker. The other contentious point is that childcare costs cannot be allowed as an expense for tax relief purposes.

Childcare, therefore, can be a highly emotive and controversial matter. However, a large number of people believe that it is wrong for mothers of young children to go out to work and that any form of childcare is an abdication of parental responsibility—although it is becoming generally more accepted as an increasing number of women do successfully combine work and family.

There is no evidence to suggest that children suffer from having substitute care, providing that the care given is warm, conscientious, stimulating and, above all, consistent. Better to have sessions of keen care from an alternative source, while a bored, frustrated mother goes to work to regain her equilibrium. It is probably true to say that happy children are the ones who have contented mothers, whether they choose to be at home or manage to fit in some work.

When greeted by retorts such as, 'What's the point of having children if you insist on continuing to work?' or 'Why have a baby if someone else is going to look after it?', it is not surprising that women do feel a measure of guilt about leaving their children. There can be days when it is hard, but it can also be heartwarming to see them happily settled with a loving carer and other children.

Family

Obviously a near relative is the cheapest and most convenient childcare option. The husband may be willing to look after the children while his nurse/wife takes on some work. For the nine to five husband, this limits nursing work to evening, weekend or night shifts, whereas a shift-working husband can be free over more general times. Husbands who are reluctant to take charge of tiny babies are probably nervous of this stage, and will probably be more at ease and willing to take care of the older child, who can enjoy swimming or walking or helping in the garden and is less likely to miss his mother.

A nearby granny may also be willing to oblige, perhaps more on an emergency basis than as a regular commitment. Young grannies are often busy themselves, having returned to work or become involved with social pursuits. Old grannies can find young children very exhausting. Most grannies can manage a few crisis days in the school holidays!

Childminder

The most likely type of paid childcare suitable for the working nurse is childminding, as a convenient, flexible, reliable and reasonably priced option.

This service has developed over the years, as the obvious answer to meet a growing need and is now assimilated into the social services. It is a legal requirement for childminders, who receive payment for caring for children under five on their own premises, to register with the correct authority. The social worker checks on amenities, hygiene and safety in the home and discusses first aid and child development. There is a limit to the number of minded children allowed at any one time and the social worker makes random visits to the household to check on the arrangement.

In the vast majority of cases, registration and inspection is a mere formality, but it is comforting to know that the service is properly organised and supervised for the wellbeing of the children. Illegal unregistered minders continue to operate, and will do for as long as mothers collude in supporting a service which can mean inferior care for a reduced price, without the guarantee of supervision.

From a list of potential minders and mums, the social worker
acts as an agent to match the requirements of each. Minders may
have a special liking for babies or a preference for older children,
they may want several children on a full-time basis or be seeking
a part-time placement.

From then on it is a private mutual arrangement between
mother and minder, who decide on details regarding payment,
hours, meals and washing. Charges are reasonable and tend to be
guided by a local rate within that area but are roughly what you
would expect to pay for a babysitter. At the negotiating stage it is
as well to have clear agreement if the minder objects to having
the child when he is ill, or, alternatively, whether you mind your
child going to the house if the minder's children are poorly. It is
also important to inquire whether she would be prepared to continue the minding arrangement during the school holidays when
her children are at home and, if you have a school child, whether
he could be included over the holidays. As minding fees come out
of one salary, it is usual for subsequent children to be charged at
half the rate of the first child.

Whatever type of arrangement you are seeking, the social
worker is bound to be able to find a minder to suit your needs. A
minder is usually a mother confined at home by the responsibility
of her own children, who is happy to earn some money by taking
in extra children. A working mother will be reassured that her
child is getting safe care by a responsible, experienced woman, in
a stimulating environment, with the possible benefit of built-in
playmates.

All it takes is a simple telephone call to the social services
department, and ask to speak to the officer responsible for childminding.

Don't forget also that if you have a friend or neighbour with
whom you might come to a childcare arrangement, why not suggest that she becomes registered, so that she can become your
minder. Someone has to make the first move and this arrangement is beneficial to both mothers. Being registered does not
compel a minder to take on any more children than she actually
wants to but it is a legal necessity, even if she only minds for payment for a few mornings per week.

Perhaps the finest accolade to childminders came from a neighbour's young child, who scowled at his mother and asked, 'Why
don't *I* have a childminder like my friend Benjy?'

Nanny

A nanny can live in or come to the house on a daily basis. She is expressly employed to look after children and will be reluctant to do domestic chores, other than those that are absolutely related to childcare.

If she is a trained general or paediatric nurse, or nursery nurse, she can expect to command a salary equal to that of a staff nurse, with any added accommodation expenses and insurance contributions.

This type of help is thorough and reliable, backed by references, but is expensive, although several children can be included in the initial outlay. It will probably be restricted to nurses who have achieved a highly paid position or whose husband can contribute to the cost, and is unlikely to be a feasible option for a nurse returning to part-time work on a modest grade of pay.

One possibility is to 'share a nanny', providing that you can find a willing nanny and another working mother. You instantly halve the fee for yourself, yet are getting good substitute childcare and a readymade companion for your child. Why not advertise in your local paper to see if you can find a suitable partner within your area, then readvertise for a nanny with your joint proposal.

Mother's help

A cheaper compromise is a mother's help, who may live in or come daily. This is a popular starter job for girls who leave school, as a way of embarking on the working world.

The mother's help is not necessarily a trained nanny, although she may be. Or she may have no experience in childcare and therefore may be of the greatest use with toddlers and older children. A mother's help can supervise children and is expected to help with some light housework and cooking, by mutual arrangement.

Au pair

An au pair is a foreign student who must have accommodation and food provided in addition to a small wage, in return for household duties and childcare or babysitting. Their childcare duties may not be sufficient to cover for a mother who goes out to work and they are not expected to be substitute mothers of young children, although they are useful to receive schoolchildren back home in the afternoon.

It may prove a satisfactory arrangement if you have room for an extra person, but there may be language difficulties, and should there be frequent changes of au pair this can disrupt the family, especially young children.

Nursery/crèche

The few local authority nurseries have long waiting lists and places are allocated by priority of need, to lone mothers or for children in deprived or disturbed circumstances.

Private nurseries are usually only equivalent to a short school day, thereby limiting a mother's job prospects which will fit around these hours. The cost will be similar to a childminder, but they rarely take children under two. Even for a child over two, it is a long tiring day and he misses the individual contact with one specific adult.

The playgroup or nursery school lasting two to three hours severely restricts commitment to any kind of job, unless a friend or childminder can collect the child and complete the day.

A crèche may be found at a workplace to cater for the children of employees. Although the health service predominantly consists of female employees, hospital crèches are surprisingly not widely available. Once again it revolves around 'politics' and availability of resources. If a health authority requires staff, it might well spend on nursery provision to attract recruits. Otherwise it will be unwilling to organise such a service when money could be diverted to other areas of overriding need. A crèche, therefore, is often a luxury which a hospital cannot afford.

To be of maximum use, any hospital crèche should run from about 7 am through until 9 or 10 pm, to span nursing shifts, but running into unsocial hours puts up the cost of service. A self-financing crèche might obviate the answer of expenditure, but that hardly helps the low-paid workers who have the outstanding need for this service.

Any hospital crèche would have to open its doors to all members of staff and not restrict it to the use of nurses, so naturally any crèche operating will be heavily oversubscribed. It is a useful childcare option to look out for, but not one that you can rely on finding.

Contingency childcare

Women captive with tiny children blithely talk about getting a job when they go to school, little realising how restricting school hours really are.

After delivering and collecting the children, add on travel time and that leaves a slim day between 9.30 am and 3 pm, and holidays occurring with profuse regularity. Then there are the bouts of sudden unforeseen and unpredictable illness, either in your own child, the childminder or her children, the nanny or a reliable granny.

These limitations encroach on the job prospects for all working women with children of school age, no less for the nurse, whose duties encompass a 24-hour service. Contingency plans need to be made for routine upheavals, not to mention advance preparations for unexpected emergencies.

If you have friends or neighbours similarly placed, you may be able to help each other out on a mutual basis, as well as building a stock of people on whom you could call. In return, be prepared to be added to *their* emergency list.

If someone is prepared to care for the children on a brief but regular basis, perhaps having them for an hour before or after school, do reward their services. Nobody minds helping out in an emergency but they do appreciate recognition for a regular responsibility. It is unfair to continually tap their good nature, when you are able to earn precisely because they *do* help out. Offer a small fee and insist, then no one feels they are obliged or being taken for granted.

The holidays present a great headache, especially the very long breaks, and your annual leave entitlement cannot possibly cover them all. Can your husband take some of his annual leave at that time? Is a granny or granny-in-law likely to be available? You may even be lucky to find a hospital that has a children's play scheme run during the holidays, often arranged on a rota system, where mothers either help out or pay for the privilege of its use.

Once again, you may find part-time working friends who would be willing to do a reciprocal swap, or a childminder keen to extend her duties to accept school-age siblings.

A mother who does not work may welcome the opportunity of some extra cash, so why not advertise on the school noticeboard for holiday help. She does not have to register as a childminder to look after children over the age of five.

Senior school pupils may also act as babysitters during the holidays. Older children are delighted by the attentions of an entertaining, buoyant teenager, who, in turn, would welcome the chance to earn some pocket money. Seek out teenagers from reliable families that you know in your neighbourhood, ask your regular babysitter or inquire at the school for a responsible person to help. Enterprising youngsters occasionally advertise their services on newsagents' boards, knowing how mothers relish some respite from continually occupying their children during the long summer holiday.

Sudden illness, not necessarily serious but sufficient to keep the child home from school, can cause a hiccough for the working mother and is something which must be thought around and planned for.

Bank and agency nurses can cancel their booked work at the last moment in such acute circumstances. A nurse on the staff may be allowed to use up annual leave to cover unexpected days off, or be able to swap a shift at short notice.

Nurse managers have discretion to allocate compassionate leave but this is reserved for serious illness, hospitalisation and deaths in close members of the family. It is for use in dire emergency only and cannot and should not be abused for minor illnesses.

At interview, it is likely that managers will wish to be reassured that a prospective nurse/mother has made suitable arrangements for her children in the holidays and in the event of illness. Although the law states that such questions which are discriminating against women may not be asked, there are ways around it. The nurse would be well advised to be prepared with suitable answers if they do arise and, if they do not, it will be assumed that arrangements have been made in anticipation of a return to work. Anyone who imposes very restrictive conditions to work may be advised to join the nurse bank scheme instead of the regular staff.

With your mind attuned to work, and practical difficulties out of the way, you are now ready to consider the possible ways in which you may return to nursing.

Reference and refresher reading

National Childbirth Trust Working Mothers Group of Clapham (1984). *The Working Mothers' Handbook—A Practical Guide to the Alternatives in Childcare.* Clapham NCT Working Mothers, 167 Fentiman Road, London SW8 1JY.

2
Welcome Back: Employment Opportunities for the Returning Nurse

Did you know that it costs around £14 000 to train a registered nurse and around £9000 to train an enrolled nurse?

In financial terms, this is a worthwhile investment if the nurse provides a substantial service to the profession by using her qualification. Should a nurse train and leave her job altogether, this cost has been a wasteful expense to the health service.

Yet, at some stage in their life, the majority of women do get married and have children, which necessitates a break in service for a variable period. Despite the opportunities that exist to allow women to stay in employment, it may not be practically feasible or emotionally desirable for an individual to retain a full-time job. If the logistics of parking one child are difficult, it becomes even more complicated and expensive for two or three!

In many families, the mother leaves her employment or cuts her hours during the early childrearing years, and will think of returning to work at a later convenient time.

So it can be expected that there are a considerable number of trained nurses who would welcome the chance to return to their career, providing it can be fitted in and around their domestic commitments and providing they can be updated to adequately fulfil their role.

In the current circumstances, a qualified nurse with a break in service of *any* length, can be re-employed as a trained nurse and virtually pick up where she left off. In theory, a nurse can legally walk back onto a ward, following an absence of 20 years, and take charge of patients, thanks to the inalienable right of the letters after her name. This is a patently absurd situation, fraught with potential dangers and one which, hopefully, will soon be remedied. It is also one which frightens the returning nurse and is an obvious and strong indication for refresher and back-to-nursing courses.

In reality, such an abrupt return to ultimate responsibility should *never* occur and no responsible employer would allow this to happen, without some prior updating and supervision of the returning nurse.

Nevertheless, a woman who is keen to return to practical nursing but is reluctant to assume the responsibility of a trained nurse, may be tempted to apply for a position as an auxiliary. Indeed, the most common lament from women contemplating a return to nursing is, 'I'd go back tomorrow if I could just work at the bedside, doing what I know best, functioning as an auxiliary, but I haven't the confidence to take charge again and I am so out of date'.

There is no legal constraint which prohibits an authority from employing a trained nurse as an auxiliary, but most are reluctant to do so and this may be written into their employment policy. It is a downright waste of useful skills and may pose an invidious situation, set to create problems amongst other staff.

Any trained nurse who is employed as an auxiliary would have to remember very carefully to act strictly within the boundaries of that capacity, and she may find this increasingly difficult as she becomes familiar with the working environment.

A request of this calibre should, however, give the impetus to hospitals to consider constructive ways of giving returning nurses the necessary help to overcome their fears and to enable them to fit back into contemporary nursing.

There is a vast pool of untapped experience in women waiting to grasp the opportunity to use their qualification and provide a useful service. Even after a break of ten years, the 35 or 40-year-old still has 25 and 20 years respectively of active nursing ahead of her. With her home settled and family completed, these should be years of uninterrupted, concentrated service, with increasing involvement in her career.

Deciding on the kind of work

The job scene makes conflicting reading because it fluctuates with time and is subject to variation in different areas of the country. On the one hand we read of 10 000 nurses on the dole, unable to find employment. Turn the page and we are told of wards closing because of insufficient staff to run the establishment.

Certainly today newly qualified nurses have no job security, and they are no longer guaranteed a post in their training hospital after successful completion of their course.

Much of the paradoxical picture of unemployment lies with the lack of mobility, resulting in mismatch of applicant and opportunity. Married women rarely have the freedom to move around chasing jobs, unless they are the breadwinner or rely on tied accommodation. Once settled, they are usually tied to a location by a combination of factors: their husband's occupation, favourable schooling and social contacts that have developed over the years. So, although they may not be able to find a suitable job close by, they are unable or unwilling to move or travel to an area where work is freely available. For the returning nurse, the ability to drive and have use of a car is an untold asset.

There are, of course, advantages in being settled in one district. As a prospective employee, you are more likely to remain for a long time in any one job or convenient place of employment than a transient youngster.

Employers will have to grasp the nettle of employing mature trained nurses and find ways of encouraging them back to the profession, which will undoubtedly involve some kind of updating and retraining.

As we approach the end of the 20th century, there is a projected decline in the population of 18-year-olds. There will be less young adults to offer themselves for basic training, and even they may be lured into other professions who will be competing for their share of the up-and-coming generation.

In the future, it is possible that the major element of care will be delivered by older married women, mature trained nurses returning as a valuable source of expert labour, providing a stable workforce for the health service.

Service managers will need to rethink how best to allocate their finite resources of money and manpower, with special consideration to current patterns of family life and work. They need to reassess that overlooked population of 'resting' trained nurses, sitting on a wealth of experience and motivation. By taking into account the domestic commitments of these women, planners need to find ways of attracting nurses back to work and making the most effective use of their service, involving back-to-nursing and refresher courses, part-time and occasional work, the provision of crèche or school holiday schemes, as well as career advancement.

Many hospitals already rely heavily on part-timers and occasional nurses, particularly for night duty and weekend work and fluctuating areas like intensive care units. Some smaller, usually rural, hospitals can function only because of a very high proportion of part-time nurses.

There is no truth in the frequently held view that part-time staff are unreliable; certainly mature people can be expected to take their responsibilities with the utmost seriousness.

Certain interesting emotions may be experienced by the nurse who returns after any absence, some of which may be disturbing to the individual or cause friction amongst staff.

Many returning nurses who are fearful of the responsibility are only too relieved that a more senior member takes ultimate charge. However, some nurses who have taken a demotion in order to work part-time for their convenience may find it hard to adjust to a junior role, having previously held a senior position.

An older woman may resent the authority of a much younger ward sister or nursing officer, of perhaps her own daughter's age. (But don't forget that the younger woman may also be finding life difficult, especially if she feels her position is threatened.)

It is equally tough to accept a blanket hospital policy which may automatically invest the position of seniority to a full-time staff nurse over a part-time, bank or agency nurse, irrespective of experience or qualifications.

Although bitchiness and bickering can still rear its head in nursing, harmony should prevail in a professional team, which acknowledges that every member has a valuable contribution to make. And being sensitive to other people's needs and feelings should be the order of the day for everyone.

Getting married women back to their career is an option, relatively cheaper and quicker than a two or three-year training. And once they are back, they are likely to stay in their jobs and probably progress further in the service.

It makes sound economic sense to utilise the skills of personnel already trained and to deploy their services when and where they are needed most. This can be achieved in a variety of ways but their availability in any area is entirely dependent on the district policy for employing nurses and the demand for staff at that particular time.

Part-time work

Part-time nurses make up a quarter to over a third of the total nursing staff in NHS hospitals, depending on what area of the UK you look at (see Figure 2.1). The trend for part-time employment for married nurses is becoming an established pattern, accepted as an efficient and frequently necessary source of trained nursing, ideal for nurse and manager alike. In the community, part-time work may also be available in school nursing, district nursing, health visiting, in a GP practice or in occupational health.

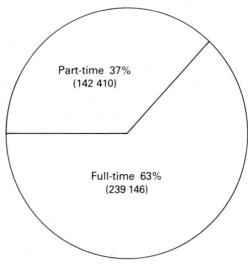

Part-time 37%
(142 410)

Full-time 63%
(239 146)

Fig. 2.1 Full-time and part-time nursing staff in the NHS, England, 1980. Taken from Salvage J. (1985). The Politics of Nursing. London: Heinemann Nursing.

Any period of employment up to 37 hours is part-time work, 37½ hours being full-time employment. Salary and holiday entitlement are both paid pro rata of the full-time rate. Sickness pay covers absence for health reasons of the employee but not for illnesses of her children. In exceptional circumstances compassionate leave may be given at the discretion of the service manager.

If a part-timer is asked to work extra hours, provided that she is still within the 37½ hour limit, she is paid at her normal rate. Yet if the hospital were to employ a full-timer to do extra hours, it would have to pay the enhanced overtime rate. So part-timers may also be used cheaply to fill in extra duties if they occur.

In general, it is far cheaper to employ nurses for exactly the time and place where they are required, rather than having a vast unnecessary overlap in the hours of least need. So, all round, part-timers give good value for money.

The likelihood of finding suitable part-time work will depend on what you have to offer, what authorities need at that precise time, how each hospital employs part-timers and how they specify terms of contract.

In times of high unemployment or NHS cutbacks, part-time jobs, together with bank nursing, agency work and back-to-nursing courses, are inevitably the first items to be trimmed. Also some hospitals may prefer to employ auxiliary staff, as a cheaper option to trained staff, especially in low-technology areas of care.

Training hospitals which have a steady throughput of learners may have limited openings for part-time nurses at any time, although there are areas where they are a cost-effective source of permanent staff. Other hospitals may require all of its nurses to work on a system of internal rotation, involving day and night duty on a set rota for each ward, so this clearly may not be possible for some married women.

The returning registered nurse will almost invariably be employed as a staff nurse, even though her pay will reflect a grade which takes account of her previous experience. Hospitals are understandably reluctant to employ nurses at a part-time sister grade, because it incurs a higher salary. However they do make exceptions in areas of notable responsibility or expertise, such as a specialist unit or taking sole charge of a small hospital at night.

Regarding part-time employment, hospitals may be happy to offer specific fixed hours for a particular area, although this is becoming less common as it restricts movement of staff around the hospital and limits flexibility of working hours. An example of fixed hours could be the evening shifts on a surgical ward for operation days, or perhaps 8 am to 1 pm each weekday to cover the busy morning period, or a fixed duty every Saturday and Sunday.

Some areas of fixed designation can occur in the outpatient department to cover specific clinics, or in a day hospital, a day surgery unit, the recovery ward attached to a theatre suite, or for some routine theatre sessions. In these areas, staff may commence work at 9 or 9.30 am, thus obviating an expensive and wasteful two hours before the clinic or theatre starts up.

Another idea is to employ a nurse for specific hours, but acting as a reserve nurse in a 'pool', to be deployed wherever she is most needed. However, this does lack continuity and possibly interferes with job satisfaction. It is probably far from ideal for the nurse returning after a long absence to be moved around in the hospital and used as an experienced nurse.

A more suitable arrangement is for the nurse to be allocated to a particular ward, employed for a set number of hours, which are fitted onto the duty rota each week to the mutual convenience of the ward and the nurse. In this situation, it is usual to expect a part-timer to take a fair share of some of the load of unsocial hours. This will be written into the contract, perhaps a commitment to one late duty per week and one weekend duty every four weeks, as an example. With the increasing number of part-timers, this is necessary to ensure that full-time staff are not penalised by getting unfairly overburdened with the unpopular shifts.

Night nurses may be employed on a fixed nights contract or for several unspecified nights, which allows some flexibility for the allocation officer and for fairer distribution of the less popular nights.

The 'unsocial hours' are so called because they conflict with the general pattern of life and interfere with social events that are enjoyed by the majority of the population who work weekdays, 9 am to 5 pm.

A hospital provides a 24-hour caring service and, by definition, requires staff to provide around-the-clock cover. Although every member of the nursing staff is expected to take a slice of these less desirable hours as a term of their employment, no one these days is expected to forfeit their outside existence by committing themselves exclusively to their job.

Unsocial hours refer to evening shifts, night duty and all work over bank holidays and weekends. Covering these hours by providing adequate staffing levels represents a constant headache for nurse managers, so that juggling with the off-duty rota is no easier than it ever was!

However, married nurses often welcome the chance to work these unsocial hours, when their built-in babysitter returns home from his job and is free to supervise the children. Too much of this can lead to a 'doorstep marriage', as partners pass on the porch, going to and from their respective places of work. Yet, a few shifts each week can benefit the family income and enhance the mother's contentment as she broadens her horizons.

As an added incentive, there is an increased rate of payment for working unsocial hours and also in some of the less popular areas of care (see page 9).

The 'twilight shift' covers evening work, possibly spanning 4 to 9 pm or 5 to 10 pm, and is a boon to a busy geriatric or surgical ward where the patients are of a high level of dependence.

At a time when the core of day staff leave, operation patients are either back, waking up and needing constant attention, or others may still need to be collected from theatre. An extra trained nurse will be of immense help with the numerous observations and infusions to check and analgesics to be given, added to the routine work, plus dealing with a stream of anxious relatives phoning and visiting.

It is useful if the twilight shift extends across the day-to-night handover, as the nurse provides some continuity of care while the night nurses take the report and get themselves organised.

Another innovative idea is the 'dawn shift'. Although it has not been widely adopted, it holds exciting prospects in areas of continuing care and rehabilitation, such as with the elderly or disabled. Rather than pay for a team of nurses to sit through the night watching the patients sleeping blissfully, one only is retained for cover. The dawn shift, from 5.30 to 8 am, arrives to assist with the bulk of the work, helping patients get washed, dressed and breakfasted, in readiness for the day's activities ahead.

These hours are eminently appealing to the larks amongst us, who are also able to be back in time to get the children off to school.

It is a popular choice for mothers to work one or two shifts over the weekend, which command a premium of higher pay.

Night duty has also always proved a popular option for the woman with children, if she is happy to adjust to alternating day and night life. Mothers can sleep in the daytime *with* tiny tots who have a nap, or *without* older children who are at school.

One night, averaging ten hours (9 pm to 8 am, with one hour mealbreak) would be equivalent to two day shifts, while paying a better rate of pay and halving transport costs.

The employment of part-time night staff is of mutual benefit. Hospitals find it hard to keep permanent full-time night nurses for any appreciable length of time. It is true to say that many hospitals depend upon steady, reliable part-timers to make up the bulk of their night nursing workforce and would be hard pressed if they had to do without the contribution made by married women.

Getting the work

Once decided on part-time work, the prospective nurse employee must plan on the number and type of hours that she can realistically manage, after close consideration of all her domestic commitments. For your own peace of mind, it is necessary to have clearly defined any childcare arrangements and contingency plans for illness and holidays. It would be an advantage if you can have a certain degree of flexibility when discussing a part-time arrangement, as a manager will look favourably on a candidate who can be accommodating to service needs.

A simple telephone inquiry to the hospital personnel or nursing department will clarify their policy regarding part-time posts and elicit if there are any vacancies currently available. You may be invited for an informal interview to discuss in general terms the possibility of employment.

Do state clearly any aspects that might be impossible, such as Sunday shifts or night work, or any areas which would give you undue concern, like working in intensive care units or being a float nurse. Say if you feel you need updating and inquire whether they run a back-to-nursing course or orientate new staff. On the other hand, be positive and enthusiastic about what you would be willing to do, especially if the manager indicates that one area of the hospital is difficult to staff and there is an urgent need for nurses.

Try not to be too restrictive, as this will limit your possibilities, but it is vital that important items are aired early on, to allow employer and employee to negotiate how best to match their requirements.

It would be foolish to commit yourself to something which is impossible to fulfil and causes problems later on. Any reasonable hospital will be understanding if you are a returning nurse with outside commitments, provided that you can keep your side of the bargain by giving a good service.

Also, do not take on more hours than you can safely work, for your health, your family and your patients! There will undoubtedly be opportunity to increase your hours at a later date, when you have proved yourself as a valuable member of the staff.

The good part-time nurse is an investment for a future full-time member of staff, and forward-thinking hospitals will aim to develop the career of part-time nurses with this end in view. All part-time nurses should be integrated with the full-time staff, to be offered incentives and training opportunities alongside their colleagues, which will enable them to keep up with changes in the profession.

If a prospective employee makes too rigid demands over her working times, she may be recommended to look for work via a nurse bank or agency.

Your local job centre will also know of nursing jobs available in the area.

Bank nursing

The idea of a hospital nursing bank has grown in popularity over recent years, as an efficient and economical way of building a reserve pool of temporary staff. A nurse may be needed to relieve staff shortage; due to sickness, during maternity leave, over holiday periods, when permanent staff go off on a course, when there is a gap in staff establishment or if a patient requires 'specialling'.

The hospital maintains a register of nurses, who state when they would be available to work. When a nurse is needed, the hospital tries to match its requirement with whoever is on the list. Duties may be booked in advance to cover foreseeable gaps, or may occur more suddenly in the event of an emergency.

This scheme benefits both the hospital and the nurse in a variety of ways.

A hospital only pays for the precise hours that the nurse is required, without paying her for a full shift with any wasteful overlap. Neither do they have to pay the expensive on-costs of staff employment—no sickness pay, no holiday pay, no superannuation, no maternity leave entitlement, no redundancy pay. Nurses count as temporary casual labour and are paid only for what they do.

Hospitals do not have to routinely employ 'float' nurses for 'just in case', when they have a source of emergency help on tap at the end of the telephone. Extra duties, that would incur an expensive overtime rate for regular full-time staff, can be allocated to a bank nurse being paid the base rate.

Hospitals interview prospective bank nurses, take up references and can select those who are suitable to go on the register. Bank nurses wear the hospital uniform and come under the jurisdiction of the hospital authority, all of which compares favourably with the 'unknown quantity' of the agency staff nurse. By employing their own staff, hospital managers largely obviate the use of agency nurses and the cost of the accompanying agency fee.

All hospitals make a great effort to support bank nurses in their role and for the nurse to feel a welcome part of the staff, with a valued contribution to the team. Many hospitals incorporate a clinical training programme, similar to a back-to-nursing course, to update older trained nurses, to motivate interest, as well as being a way of controlling standards and delivery of care. Indeed, it is considered unwise to appoint nurses directly to clinical practice unless they have been well orientated to current methods in use.

Nurses may be recruited to the nurse bank, following completion of the hospital's back-to-nursing course. Understanding authorities may permit returning nurses to limit their level of responsibility initially, until the nurses build up their confidence and current knowledge. It is obvious that bank nurses are a likely source of staff for the permanent establishment in the future when the nurse can commit herself to more work.

Nurse banks comprise women who are unable to undertake full-time work or a job on a regular part-time basis, perhaps because a husband does shift work or frequently travels away on business. It is also ideal for the mother who would have difficulty with childcare supervision in the holidays or in the event of sudden illness.

Although a bank nurse has stated beforehand when she is available, the nurse can refuse a duty without jeopardising future opportunities, because managers realise how difficult it can be for mothers to make the necessary arrangements at short notice.

By the same token, the disadvantage is that the nurse cannot be guaranteed work, even though she is available. Neither has she any job security. A bank exists to serve any current need for staff but would close if the hospital was up to its quota on funded establishment. The bank is vulnerable in times of economic stringency.

Working on an irregular basis, through the bank, a nurse must expect to be flexible and she may find she is allocated to any—indeed every—hospital department on a random basis as the need arises. She is likely to be moved around, to be asked to check drugs and relieve meal breaks, so she may miss the continuity of one ward location. But most nurses accept this as an inevitable situation as regards this form of employment, and take it as part and parcel of being able to fit in any work at all.

Alternatively, a nurse may find she is assigned to one particular ward or unit, with which she becomes totally familiar and this is good for ward continuity and her job satisfaction. Indeed, she may find that her services come to be relied upon, to the extent where she virtually joins the permanent staff and is fitted into their duty list each week by prior arrangement.

A qualified nurse is paid at the appropriate salary scale, which takes past service into account. National insurance contributions are deducted at source but the bank nurse is expected to deal with tax payments individually with her tax officer.

Joining a nurse bank is an excellent way to keep in touch with the work scene, with the profession, maintaining links and preserving confidence, for the nurse who must leave full-time employment. It also provides a gentle reintroduction for the nurse returning to work after a long absence. Some full-time nurses may also offer their services via a bank when they are wanting to do extra work and earn extra money.

For the returning nurse, the bank gives the opportunity to gradually build up the hours that she chooses to work. Also, she is ideally placed, on site and well known for her past contribution, to apply for a permanent part-time or full-time post on the staff, when family circumstances allow.

Hospitals in both the NHS and the private sector may be operating a bank nurse scheme. Telephone the nursing office or personnel office of your local hospital to see if they run a scheme to which you may apply, or look through your local paper where they may be advertising for staff.

Agency nursing

A nursing agency is an employment agency, licensed by the local borough council, to match clients requiring nurses with nurses who are seeking a job.

The client may be a hospital or nursing home in either the NHS or private sector, it could be an individual needing care at home or to be 'specialled' in hospital, or the client could be an institution, perhaps wanting a residential school nurse or occupational health nurse.

Nurses with any type of qualification can be found jobs, while untrained personnel (including learners working in their time off!) will be employed in an auxiliary capacity. References are taken up for all those joining the agency.

The nurse is expected to provide and launder her own uniform. Some larger agencies have adopted their own uniform, and try to encourage its use by nurses in their employ.

Weekly wages are calculated from a fixed basic hourly rate for either staff nurse, enrolled nurse or auxiliary grade. Although the rate is slightly higher than the NHS to start with, they take no account of experience and there are no annual incremental rises to look forward to. Certain specialties attract a higher rate of basic pay, as does night duty, weekend and bank holiday work. The agency is required to deduct national insurance contributions and income tax on earnings that exceed the minimum tax and national insurance free limit. Nurses can choose to work sufficient hours that will not incur these expenses.

The duration of jobs may consist of odd shifts to relieve an emergency or cover an unexpected absence, or it may be in the temporary nature of a week or two, or a fairly permanent post, when the nurse is added to the regular staff roster. The type of work offered may be extremely diverse and varied, stretching across the whole spectrum of possible expertise required of a qualified nurse.

At home, an elderly lady might want a nurse as a virtual companion and aid, or a convalescent person may like the assurance of a trained nurse on the premises. In hospital, the nurse may be wanted as an extra pair of hands in a busy area or she might be expected to take charge of a ward. At the other end of the spectrum of care, a patient may require intensive care on a ventilator, with drips, drains, monitors and a plethora of observations, following trauma or delicate surgery. In the London area in particular there appears to be a preponderance of jobs in the specialty areas of intensive care units (ICU); coronary care units (CCU), special care baby units (SCBU), and theatre work, all of which require a high ratio of nurses in constant supply.

Nurses are quite at liberty to state a preference for the work they undertake, many choosing only to work in the area with which they are totally familiar.

So, with a wide range of opportunities available, the returning nurse can expect to be *offered* a huge selection of vacancies, some of which may be patently beyond her capability in the initial stages.

Remember, that for a flexible, resourceful nurse, well versed and up to date in modern nursing, a rapid change of jobs may provide an interesting and stimulating challenge. It does, however, take considerable confidence and versatility to take charge of 28 surgical patients at night, in an unfamiliar hospital, with whose particular routine, layout and policies you are not acquainted! Such a situation could impose an unacceptable strain on a newly returned nurse, already struggling to keep pace with her designated role and updating herself with current practice.

If you can attend any type of refresher course within the locality prior to joining an agency, this will widen your horizons in the nursing world and build your confidence.

The key to successful and beneficial employment via an agency is to state explicitly what type of work you are willing to undertake and to be prepared to refuse some opportunities that are beyond your scope at present. Always check the details of any job on offer and find out just what your position would entail.

Any client who employs you will do so on the assurance that the agency, in good faith, is sending a nurse fully competent to fulfil the stated obligation. Any responsible agency, keen to maintain its good reputation with a client, will be equally anxious to send the right nurse for the right job. It is an unscrupulous agency that tries to persuade a nurse to bluff her way through a job for which she feels incapable or in an area of care in which she is unsure of practice. *Never* be coerced into accepting a job that you feel is outside your current capabilities. It is neither fair to you, nor the employing authority, nor the patients in your care.

There should, however, be no problem in securing suitable work for the returning nurse. An agency with a good relationship with a hospital, can easily explain your situation, your reservations about intensive care units and taking charge, and they may be happy to place you in a less demanding area of care. They will be grateful to have been warned and you can accept the job in the full knowledge that they are prepared to make allowances for your current limitations. As your experience grows, so will your confidence, and your ability to take on a wider scope of duties.

Agency work is convenient because it allows you to choose the amount of work you do in periods when you are most freely available. You may opt to work in term time and be free in the school holidays. But be warned, there are a limited number of jobs available for the 9 am to 3 pm period, so you may need childcare for an early or late overlap.

Another good advantage is that you can get an inside view of a local hospital or nursing home, which may be useful for future consideration. By working there, you will get a feedback on the atmosphere, together with a good idea of the workload and staff situation. A good agency nurse who fits in may well be invited to join the permanent staff should a position become available.

To find a nursing agency in your area, look under the small ads of the local newspaper or in the yellow pages telephone directory. Contact agencies initially to inquire which hospitals or homes they serve, as travel may be a factor for you to consider. Go and discuss the possibility of employment, considering your absence, and judge for yourself whether they will handle this situation reasonably and be prepared to be helpful to you. Do state at the outset exactly what you would be willing to undertake and what you could *not* manage.

You may register with several agencies to improve your chances of suitable work, although the agencies would not endorse this.

A general nurse returning to nursing via an agency after a ten-year absence said:

> I was nervous to return at first and careful about the jobs I took. But, after a few weeks on the wards, everything fell easily into place and it was as if I'd never been away.

Non-NHS employment

The recent growth in the private sector has thrown open the market for more nursing jobs, which may be of varying interest and availability to the returning nurse.

A private institution is unlikely to organise a back-to-nursing course, unless motivated by a pressing need for staff. However, most do provide a substantial orientation period to all new nurses joining their staff, who may spend time both as observers and as shadows to an established nurse. It is easy to see how this type of gentle and sympathetic introduction to newcomers could be extended to involve those returning after a period of absence from nursing. You may be asked to do your observation in an unpaid capacity but this is a small price to pay for the chance to get reacquainted with your profession, with the promise of a job when you become confident and proficient.

The director of nursing would consider each job applicant on individual merit. It would be at her discretion to employ a returning nurse, largely based on the candidate's training, past experience and the result of references, all taken into account with the length of absence. In a personal interview, the director could gauge the temperament of the person, how adaptable she is likely to be, if she could take to new situations and assimilate into that particular organisation. Much would depend on the type of work in the institution, their current need for trained staff and whether suitable arrangements could be made for the nurse to be guided and supervised into a viable position of employment, together with the disposition of the person.

Private hospitals that concentrate on acute care, some of which includes highly specialised surgery, rely exclusively on trained nurses who can shoulder the responsibility of the full range of patient care. Qualified nurses have a unique position of autonomy, a high level of accountability, are expected to make their own decisions and often required to relate directly with the patient's consultant. Nurses may like the one-to-one nurse/patient relationship of caring for people in single rooms, but they are expected to be on their toes and have the utmost confidence to act on their own responsibility, which takes considerable courage. On a general surgical floor, the nurse would need to be clinically up to date to cope with the variety of cases, from ENT to gynaecology, from bowel surgery to dental extraction.

As private hospitals have no auxiliary help or learners, the nurse can miss out on the comforting support of other staff working with her, although of course no nurse would be left alone until the director was satisfied that she could cope. Mature nurses are also often more ready to accept the finer niceties of the hotel services demanded by those in private care.

Private hospitals will often organise a nurse bank, to have a pool of trained staff at their disposal, or use agency staff if necessary.

In the more leisurely, less technical environment of a home for the elderly, the convalescent or the chronic sick, where the pace is slower and geared to basic care and rehabilitation, the returning nurse may find her niche. It is likely that an employer would look favourably on the returning nurse, who has retained the fundamental nursing skills and has a mature, stable outlook on life. This type of working situation may be an attractive proposition to both parties.

The private sector pays marginally better than the NHS and may provide other incentives, such as uniform, subsidised meals on duty, pension and private health insurance.

There is no shortage of private institutions in and around the London area, and other big cities are also served well now. In areas that attract retired people, there is usually a proliferation of private homes for the elderly, especially on the South Coast, which has been aptly named 'the Costa Geriatrica'.

To find available private institutions in your area, consult the yellow pages telephone directory, listing hospitals and nursing homes. You could also ask at the local health centre, the social services department, the community health council or the district health authority offices. An easier method is to phone a local nursing agency and ask which private institutions regularly use their services.

If you telephone or write to the director of nursing (still often called the matron, especially in nursing homes) and explain your situation and proposal, she will undoubtedly suggest an informal interview to discuss the possibility of employment. As private organisations are invariably smaller than those in the NHS, you will be able to get the personal attention of the top person. Being attuned to good public relations, she will undoubtedly give a fair-minded assessment of your offer and be in a position to make suitable arrangements within her organisation.

Voluntary work

A veritable army of volunteers provides an admirable service for the sick, elderly and disabled in a number of ways, delivered by three major avenues: in hospital, in the community and through charity organisations.

Any voluntary work has a dual benefit, as it not only helps those in need, but provides a useful, fulfilling and altruistic outlet for the helpers. Although unpaid, it is an ideal way of being involved with other people, having an interest beyond the home, feeling good about doing a helpful task, as well as generally boosting confidence and making use of hidden or rusty talents.

Numerous charities and voluntary agencies—such as Dr Barnardo's, National Children's Home, Mencap, Help the Aged—rely upon a wide network of voluntary help to support their causes. For fund-raising, they require helpers in their charity shops, for street collections or to sell cards and gifts from their mail order catalogue.

Direct practical help is needed when charities organise outings and they depend on assistance with transportation, wheeling the chairbound or joining with the handicapped on sports events or swimming.

The community services call upon volunteers to give an extra dimension to the lives of the housebound and elderly, who might otherwise lead a difficult and isolated existence. There is a limit to what a professional employee can offer to each individual, when she has many clients on her casebook with pressing needs.

The volunteer can give help in a variety of ways at a leisurely pace: driving an old lady to a dental appointment, to the library or the hairdressers, shopping, granny-sitting to relieve a single carer, writing letters or reading to the elderly, or simply providing regular companionship for a lonely person. 'Task Force' is an organisation which coordinates volunteers to give help to the elderly with chores such as gardening, decorating and spring cleaning.

Some nurse/mothers find a special affinity with those organisations concerning mothers and babies, like the National Childbirth Trust (NCT) or Baby Life Support Systems (BLISS). These are a natural combination of their nursing talents and newly found motherhood, with the overwhelming advantage that babies and toddlers are accepted in the background of activities.

From a wide selection of tasks required in the locality, the volunteer can choose the type of help to give, at times which best fit in with her domestic commitments. Most boroughs run a coordinating agency, in order to deploy help wisely and rationally, endeavouring to match what the helper can offer to the person who could make use of it.

To find out how you may offer your services for voluntary help, make inquiries at either the library, the social services department, the civic centre or the Citizen's Advice Bureau (CAB).

Voluntary work in hospital

The most logical placement for the nurse/volunteer is to join the estimated quarter of a million people who regularly help in hospitals.

Their services may be organised through a League of Hospital Friends or appointed to a nursing officer who will allocate and supervise their positions. In big hospitals that accrue a large and varied volunteer workforce, a voluntary service coordinator (VSC) may be engaged to get volunteers gainfully deployed to the areas of need, who request particular services.

The Women's Royal Voluntary Service (WRVS) operate in about 1000 hospitals nationwide, and the Red Cross Society offer a selection of welfare activities, including a beauty/make-up/manicure service to patients.

The voluntary role is for patient comforts only and must be careful not to encroach on jobs that would threaten to deprive a paid worker of his livelihood. So, although voluntary work is strongly endorsed, willingly given and gladly received, helpers must not be utilised as free, alternative staff. Volunteer resources complement the staff, and never act as substitutes.

Nevertheless, there are a whole host of useful tasks awaiting hospital volunteers, to contribute to the welfare of patients, relatives and staff. They may run errands or help feed patients, arrange flowers, entertain children to give the parents a welcome break, or be involved in clerical jobs. Other work includes taking around the trolley shop and library trolley, acting as an escort, hairdressing, manning the outpatient department canteen or hospital radio, plus the multitude of chores involved in the smooth execution of the annual bazaar. There is something for everyone, from teenagers to pensioners!

Two cardinal sins must be avoided when volunteers are allocated to a ward or department. The first sin, indeed an insult, is to leave a volunteer idle, letting her feel that her offer of help has been wasted. Nothing disposes of a volunteer faster than making her feel either unwelcome or that she is a nuisance, whose presence is really more of a hindrance than a help.

The second sin is to abuse the person's offer by exploitation or by expecting them to undertake distasteful or stressful tasks, which they are not prepared to do. All volunteers are most willing, yet some may be very scared of hospitals, worse still of being asked to do something unsavoury or beyond their capabilities. Tasks should be interesting, suited to individual volunteers, have an obvious value, yet not be intimidating or offputting.

A nurse/volunteer would be a welcome asset to a ward as she would not flinch at rolling up her sleeves and getting closely involved with patient care if requested. This, however, may be an abhorrent suggestion to one whose idea of voluntary help is clearly restricted to work in the hospital shop or fundraising.

The nurse offering herself as a volunteer will need to remain within the confines of a volunteer's duty but is ideally placed to observe the comings and goings of hospital life. Just being in and around the clinical milieu can be one step closer to the work situation, an opportunity to 'test the water' of the employment scene in safety. You become acquainted with the caring service, of either the community or the hospital and refresh yourself as to the needs of the sick person.

Being on hand to chat with staff enables you to estimate the likelihood of work prospects and to ask if they run any refresher courses.

It also offers the chance to see how easily you can fit work hours around your domestic responsibilities. Commitment by intention, rather than contract, can be severed without trauma to either party, if adverse circumstances affect the situation.

Once back in the familiar hospital environment, most nurses are surprised at how comfortable they soon feel. They regain their confidence and everything slots back into place with ease, as they become reassured about their ability to offer themselves once again into a real nursing role.

If you are still unsure of the skills and expertise that you possess, sit back and take a hard look at what you have to offer.

3

What Have You Got to Offer?

It will probably come as no surprise to learn that women, when emerging from a period of domesticity and asked to assess their attributes, have the invariable tendency to underestimate themselves. Modesty, together with a lack of assertiveness, seems to dictate that women list their weaknesses before their strengths.

Take any woman who has been at home with young children for several years and ask her how she views the prospect of returning to work. The usual threefold answer will comprise, 'I'm out of touch, out of date and have lost my confidence'. This applies whether she is a hairdresser envisaging modern styles, a secretary faced with new office technology or a nurse or teacher having to contend with new methods, ideas and equipment.

Unfortunately, commencing with a negative stance creates a barrier to progress, both mentally and physically. The negative aspects assume such frightening magnitude that they quickly overshadow all those positive and valuable assets that the woman has to offer. If she concentrates and persists with all the things she 'can't do' and 'doesn't know', she will never give herself the chance to realise all the positive aspects on her side, thereby reinforcing and accelerating the downward spiral of self-worth and self-confidence.

No nurse should be allowed to underrate the skills and talents which she has attained, and will find she has retained, once given the opportunity to practise again. Manipulative skills, such as learning to swim, drive a car or ride a bike, can quickly be regained even after a period of inactivity. Any nurse, even in a two or three-year basic training period will have mastered, perfected and repeated a wide variety of practical techniques that can easily be polished up in the right circumstances. Think how proficient you had become with giving injections, passing a nasogastric tube and doing untold numbers of dressings. You could do that again tomorrow, if asked.

Much of the basic knowledge you learned must also be hidden

there in the recesses of your mind. Even if it does seem dormant at present, that is only because you have not had occasion to use it, but it can be quickly summoned forward, to be built upon as required. You have a valuable fund of knowledge about the human body, what happens when it goes wrong and how it can be treated.

Nursing is always with you, because it is so fundamental to everyday life. Not many nurses manage to avoid being called upon as the casual adviser for ailments within their neighbourhood; whether it be children's cuts, bumps, spots or fevers or the adult with a sprain, fracture or a coronary, it all counts for using your knowledge and experience.

The involvement with hospital life and nursing work is never wasted, and a basic training is a useful asset in itself when applying for non-nursing work. But, imagine how comfortable you feel in a clinical setting; you know the routine, the layout, the staff roles and can understand the jargon. As you walk along a hospital corridor, you know what is meant by ECG, EEG, ANC, A and E, pathology and haematology. If your relative is admitted, you understand the terms D and V, ENT, HNPU and would know what to expect when blood is taken, an examination performed or an infusion set up. In brief, you are familiar with the environment and know the ropes, which should give you a head start over learners who have to assimilate all of this peripheral knowledge.

In your past working life you have to your credit hundreds of patients in your care, having dealt with a wide variety of physical conditions, personalities and problems, both great and small. Can you recall how two of you managed a ward throughout the night, how you 'specialled' a particular patient and how you coped with the unknown quantity of the casualty department?

Do you ever think back to a situation that you felt you had handled poorly as a student at the age of 18, knowing full well that your management of it would be significantly better if faced with it again tomorrow? Certainly, there are a lot of other assets that you will have gained from those extra years of general experience of life and much will have come from having to cope with the responsibility of a home and growing children. Do not think of it as wasted time. Most of all, do not undervalue to either yourself or others, your experience as a housewife, mother or any voluntary work, as well as all that you have learned in the 'university of life'. Employers, patients and nursing colleagues are quick to recognise and appreciate the talents brought to the clinical situation by the older nurse. Mothers learn to struggle through the next day, when children have kept them awake half the night, whereas a younger girl might sink to her knees with exhaustion!

The advantages of maturity

Under the blanket heading of maturity, here is a list of some of the assets the older woman is likely to have gained during her stay at home:

- tolerance and stamina
- tenacity and fortitude
- tact and diplomacy
- skill with personal relationships
- ability to listen and give wise counsel
- confidence to talk on sensitive matters
- organisational skills of managing a home and the finances
- personal experience of pregnancy, childbirth, sick children, possibly elderly parents and bereavement.

Returning nurses, who themselves may be struggling to regain their confidence and become up to date, can feel terribly intimidated by the young nurses abounding with theory and brimming with knowledge. But nursing theory has to be reinforced by clinical practice and students have much to learn by example from the more mature nurse, who has that experience and understanding on her side.

If you worry that there is a lot of new technology to master, rest assured that there are feelings and emotions to be handled that are as old as time and never change. Pain, anxiety, depression, discomfort, fear, sorrow and anguish are pressing problems for the patient requiring swift and competent alleviation or support. The management of fine human emotions and situations may rest more easily on the shoulders of older people, whose judgements may be better accepted as the authoritative word.

Patients may prefer to speak to a married nurse about marital or sexual problems. Teenage patients often find it difficult to talk freely to a nurse of the same age about personal matters and may seek out a mother figure.

Age tempers your own emotions and responses and tends to put a different perspective on some aspects of life. This is particularly evident as regards interpersonal relationships amongst the staff. A young nurse who may be very upset at being spoken to harshly or corrected about her work is likely to react quite differently 20 years later, with wisdom and self-assurance for support. They are not inclined to take 'bitchy' problems to heart and can manage to cope with the 'difficult' people with whom everyone finds they work at some time or another. Returning nurses, whose memories are of quaking with fear as matron did her round, find they are no longer overawed by senior nurses when they resume employment.

It is, of course, fair comment to say that a ward or department benefits from having a good cross-section of staff members, of different ages, levels of knowledge and experience. Senior staff feed from the stimulation of enquiring learners, who in turn can gain a lot from their more experienced colleagues.

However, there are certain practical assets of the mature nurse which do not escape the notice of employers. A married woman who has completed her family and has her roots settled in the district, is a fairly secure prospect for firm future employment. If she likes her job and is given opportunity for professional development the chances are that she will increase her hours as domestic responsibilities allow, and she will rejoin the career ladder staying within the locality, indeed, a captive employee, unlike a younger unattached nurse whose role may be affected by a number of variables—job mobility, the lure of marriage, relocation of domicile, pregnancy.

Mature nurses are notably reliable, conscientious, sensible and, apart from true emergencies, not distractable. For the working mother, her time out of the house at work *is* her distraction from everyday home life.

Nurses are not alone in feeling trepidation about returning to their profession. The cornerstone to success is to capitalise on your talents and to realise that the move to updating is not as difficult as you might imagine. Moreover, if you carefully scrutinise your life, you will find you have much to offer.

It is useful to take the time to work through the following morale-boosting exercise. By taking stock and making a positive assessment of your attributes, you should be greatly encouraged to see before you a wide range of capabilities.

Think positive point strategy

Choose a quiet uninterrupted half-hour, get seated comfortably with a cup of tea and pencil and paper at hand. Concentrate your mind, think back hard and pull the facts from hibernation, as you work through this exercise.

- Make a list of the areas of work to which you were allocated, during your training and in subsequent experiences, not forgetting the wards, departments, night duty, secondments and special units.
- Choose one of those areas and think briefly through the day or night routine and of the tasks in which you were involved, together with the types of conditions affecting patients in that area.
- Think of one particular patient and try to list the elements of nursing involved in his or her care.
- Try to outline briefly both the circulatory and renal systems.
- Make a list of the routine preparation of a patient prior to a general anaesthetic.
- Make a list of instructions for a patient with a newly applied plaster of Paris.
- Could you teach a learner the care of a patient following surgery and the possible complications involved in the post-operative period?
- List all the other assets you have gained during your period at home and remember to capitalise on any community activities you have been associated with, such as National Childbirth Trust, toddler club, parent–teacher associations, charity work, the Brownies, Sunday school, extra reading or evening classes, or other studies.

This exercise should make you feel a lot better. Don't fear that nursing has changed *so* dramatically. The essential core to the basic nurse training remains constant and those added frills and skills of contemporary care can be assimilated with relative ease. Younger nurses tend to get very wrapped up and carried away by the fascinating technical aspects of the work and it is often left for the experienced nurse to remember the 'little' things which count towards patient comfort and contentment—tender loving care (TLC) at the bedside.

Curriculum vitae

It is useful to collate the previous information into some kind of order, which will provide you with a permanent reference about yourself and your career pattern.

A curriculum vitae (CV) is the biographical sketch of one's working life, giving a clear idea of your background, training, qualifications and experience to any potential employer. Once you have prepared your CV, it is beneficial to have it presented well by a good typist, who can produce it with an attractive layout. Then get some photocopies made for future use and to accompany job applications.

Although much of the information will need to be duplicated onto a standard job application form, a CV provides a useful reference for events long past, and can be sent with initial letters of general inquiry.

A CV should include the following details, set out as in Figure 3.1 (see pages 50–1):

- name, including maiden or previous names, as previous employment may be recorded in these
- age and date of birth
- dependants, children and older relatives
- home address and telephone number, including STD code
- mention a current clean driving licence, if your job is likely to require this
- qualifications, dates attained and institution of training course (a) academic, 'O' and 'A' levels, diplomas, degrees, and (b) professional, and both should include grades or special merit awards attained
- courses, any of which are relevant to work, such as Art of Examining or management
- publications, in books or magazines
- a list of previous employments with dates, in chronological order
- outside pursuits, especially anything which denotes how you have retained an interest in your profession and in community activities.

CURRICULUM VITAE

Mrs Jane TAYLOR (née ALLINSON)
Age: 40   Date of birth:1–9–1946
Married   Three children aged 14, 12, 10
36, Frognall Road, Marsdale, ALTONSHIRE
Tel: 086–32–5916
I possess a clean, current driving licence and own a car.

Qualifications
Academic
1962   6 GCE 'O' levels   English language (3) English literature (3) French (6) Chemistry (4) History (2) Human Biology (1)
(Halston Grammar School)

1964   2 GCE 'A' levels   English language (3) Biology (3)
(Halston Grammar)

1968   1 AEB 'A' level   Sociology (grade C)
(Halston Polytechnic)

Professional
1967   SRN   Portsea General Hospital, HALSTON.
1969   ONC (Hons)   Knobhill Orthopaedic Hospital, HALSTON
1971   Part A Dip. Nurs.   Marsdale College of Further Education, MARSDALE

Courses
1970   Art of Examining Course   Marsdale General Hospital
1984   Back to Nursing Course   Marsdale General Hospital

Publications
1970   Care Study in the *Nursing Times*

Previous Employment
1964–1967   SRN training. Portsea General Hospital, HALSTON
1967–1968   Staff Nurse, Gynaecology Ward. Portsea General Hospital

1968–1969	ONC training. Knobhill Orthopaedic Hospital, HALSTON
1969–72	Sister. Professorial Orthopaedic Unit. Marsdale General Hospital
1972–1974	Part-time Clinical Teacher (18 hours). Marsdale General Hospital
1984–1986	Bank Nurse (average 20 hours per week). Marsdale General Hospital

Outside Activities

| 1975–1979 | Postnatal support group leader. Marsdale National Childbirth Trust |
| 1981–1984 | Volunteer helper at Swithin's Home for the Elderly. PTA Chairperson |

Fig. 3.1 A sample curriculum vitae.

Job application

It is perfectly acceptable to make a tentative enquiry to the personnel department or nursing office, to clarify whether there is any possibility of available work to suit your requirements and qualifications.

You may telephone to see if it is worth further pursuing work in a particular institution. If you choose to send an initial 'on spec' letter, it is obvious that it should look neat and tidy, to create a good first impression. Make a practice copy to get the layout correct, and write a brief, simple letter on plain notepaper, in your best handwriting. State if you are responding to an advertisement that you saw in a national magazine or the local paper.

If you address a letter to a named person, Dear Miss Jones, then you sign, 'yours sincerely', but if it is to an unknown person, Dear Sir or Madam, then you sign 'yours faithfully'. (Remember, you never have two 's's'—Sir and sincerely.)

With a brief letter of introduction and enquiry, it would be useful to attach a copy of your CV, to give details at a glance of your past experience.

You may be invited to make an informal visit to discuss the prospect of work, and this enables both prospective employer and employee to find out more about each other without any

52 *Back to Nursing with Confidence*

commitment. It will be important to discuss factors related to
your family life, such as weekend or night duty, or related to your
professional life, if you would feel unsure of being allocated to any
particular area. You may also want to ask about salary or accommodation, if this is required.

On an informal visit, you have the opportunity to look around
your place of prospective employment and perhaps meet those
people with whom you would be working. This may colour your
decision, either positively or negatively, as to whether to go
ahead with a formal application for a position.

When you are sent an application form, this will require similar information that can be copied from your CV. It is always
advisable to practise filling in the details on a separate sheet of
plain paper, to ensure that the original final copy will be carefully
completed, unspoiled and perfect.

All job applications require references to follow up, one from a
recent employer or, in the case of a long absence of a nurse, a previous employer and the training school. A second reference may
be required from a responsible citizen who knows you well, for
what is often called a 'character reference', such as the vicar, your
health visitor or a neighbour with a position of good standing in
the community. Although previous employers are in the habit of
giving references and expect to do so for their workers, it is
common courtesy that the permission of those giving personal
references is asked before they are named. When making this
simple request, it is useful to explain the exact nature of the job
which you are seeking, so that the person may gauge and word
his reference favourably and pertinently. For example, if you
were going for a job as a mountain-climbing instructor, the ref-
eree would say you had a good head for heights and a steady
hand and good nerve, but for a job as a staff nurse on a geriatric
unit he would incline his reference to attributes of patience, understanding and a genuine interest in the welfare of old people.

Together with your application form, you may be sent a copy
of the job description, which clarifies the elements of that particular role, as shown in Figure 3.2.

It is worth remembering that a well-presented, clearly written
application form and CV will put the interview panel in a recep-
tive frame of mind. It is very distracting and offputting to have to
plough through hard-to-decipher handwriting or a paper that
looks careless and messy, thus creating an impression of disorder

JOB DESCRIPTION

Title of Post: Staff Nurse
Accountable to: Ward Sister

Purpose and Duties

(A) *Purpose*

To maintain a high standard of patient care at all times.

To supervise nurses in training. To participate in ward management.

To liaise with Medical Staff in other Departments within the Hospital.

(B) *Duties*

1. To allocate duties to nurses and work with them so as to ensure that patients receive the prescribed treatment and nursing care.
2. To support the Ward Sister and deputise for her in her absence.
3. To attend ward rounds with medical staff, as required.
4. To maintain good working relationships with colleagues, medical staff and other paramedical colleagues in order to ensure good patient care.
5. To participate in full implementation of individualised patient care (Nursing Process) and to take part in clinical teaching.
6. To participate in programmes arranged for in-service training.
7. To participate in implementation of agreed Health and Safety and Fire policies. To report all accidents, incidents and complaints to the Ward Sister.
8. To apply and see that junior staff apply standards of nursing care, as agreed with the Ward Sister.
9. To maintain patients' records in accordance with agreed policies.
10. To ensure that agreed procedures pertaining to drugs and complex nursing procedures are strictly adhered to.

Continued

11. To participate in the exchange of information between night and day staff to ensure good individualised patient care.

12. To see that equipment is used effectively and economically and is suited to requirements.

13. To order as required (maintaining safe but economical stock levels) of linen, drugs and other supplies. To report discrepancies to Ward Sister.

14. To apply agreed procedures for maintaining contacts appropriate to the ward, in particular, dealing with relatives and visitors; reporting difficulties to the Ward Sister.

Fig. 3.2   An example of the job description for a staff nurse's post (from St Vincent's Orthopaedic Hospital, Pinner, Middlesex).

and lack of interest. If there are several applicants for one job, interviewers may have to evaluate from a lot of paperwork. Their view of you may be prejudiced if they are considering your application initially on the written material that you have sent.

Interview

If you are called for interview, do reply to acknowledge that you are able to attend at the specified date and time, so they will know to expect you. Should the date or time be unavoidably difficult, do telephone immediately, to explain your predicament, in the hope that they can make another appointment. As it is quite a task to assemble an interview panel within a hospital, it is best that you make every effort to attend when it suits them.

A formal interview panel will assess how suitable you are likely to be for the job they have to offer. They will have gained a thumbnail sketch of your potential from the application form, which is planned to ask most of what they require to know, but a conversation will obviously allow them to learn more about you as an individual.

It goes without saying that your interview attire should be smart and comfortable, as employers do take notice of grooming and presentation.

If you are applying for a special post in a particular type of nursing, it is necessary to do some homework about that role and that area of care. It would obviously be useful to read the nursing press over the previous few months and consult a specialty text-book, to have a workable understanding of current ideas. Show your enthusiasm and be prepared to talk about why you want that particular job and what you feel you could contribute. 'Yes' or 'no' answers give a poor indication of your personal attributes or motivation. On the other hand, it is not necessary to drone on at length beyond what is asked of you.

It is perfectly in order to state your limitations due to a period of absence from nursing, but you should demonstrate your will-ingness to learn and become updated. Be confident about your achievements and what you have to offer, as your past experience is of great value. At interview it is also reasonable to ask about opportunities for professional development and mention your own career ambitions.

You will be invited to ask questions, so take the opportunity to ask anything you feel you need to know about the job or employ-ment in general, hours of duty, salary and proposed date of com-mencement if successful. Do mention if you have a holiday already booked, as this will undoubtedly be honoured, even if you have not yet earned enough annual leave.

Your interview may also include a medical assessment in the occupational health department, to determine your fitness for employment, and will comprise questioning about your past and present health in confidence.

Do not necessarily expect to be told at interview if your appli-cation has been successful. Very often employers reserve the right to communicate their decision by letter. If you have been success-ful and are offered the job, with a starting date, you must reply straightaway with a letter to confirm that you accept the post.

4

Preparation for the Returning Nurse

As the situation stands currenly, any trained nurse may return to employment in the capacity of a qualified nurse, on the strength of her qualification, irrespective of the date when she trained or when she last worked. There is no standardised course of preparation devised for nurses who wish to return to their career after a substantial absence.

In 1987, when the UKCC plan to introduce periodic licensing for trained nurses, every nurse in current practice should be involved in regular updating schemes of continuing education. Any authority wishing to employ returning nurses, whose involvement in revision programmes had lapsed during her absence, would be expected to provide adequate refresher and updating instruction. This would need to be geared to each nurse in consideration of her break in service and would be tailored to local policy and the proposed area of work situation (see page 87).

This should, of course, apply at present, even though there is no statutory responsibility to do so. However, it is obviously in the best interests of the health authority to ensure that each nurse is a safe and competent practitioner in contemporary nursing and will, therefore, make the appropriate arrangements. This may be achieved either through a back-to-nursing course, a refresher course or an induction course when the nurse commences work.

If no such course is available in your area, there are various other stratagems which would enable the resting nurse to stimulate her interest and maintain links with her profession.

Back-to-nursing course

Because there is no statutory requirement to provide any retraining for the returning nurse, back-to-nursing courses will be arranged at the discretion of individual health authorities, sub-ject to their need to recruit staff. They are established and funded to attract new nurses and will be designed to suit the require-ments of hospitals within that district.

There is no reliable way of estimating the number of back-to-nursing courses running at any one time in the country, as they spring up and die down, as staff requirements fluctuate. Hospi-tals that are well-staffed and have plenty of learners, both as cur-rent workers and prospective qualified staff, will be unlikely to run such a course. This is probably true of most teaching hospi-tals, particularly those in London.

Alternatively, for smaller, rural hospitals, who often rely on the services of the nurse/mother working part-time, a regular back-to-nursing course may be an important aid to generating the interest of potential recruits in the locality. Courses will be advertised in the local paper, in the library or on noticeboards in shops and health centres, to seek out and attract resting qualified nurses.

The way in which a course is organised will depend on the availability of teaching staff and clinical areas, as well as reflect-ing the needs of the course members. Members may have had an absence of between two and 25 years (average is ten), with ages ranging from 23 to 50 in any group, each presenting with varying domestic commitments.

The aims of a back-to-nursing course are five-fold:

- to revise practical skills and introduction of new methods, with guided supervision of practice.
- to reinforce and update the role of the professional nurse in current practice.
- to orientate nurses to hospital departments, personnel and local health services.
- to instil confidence in the potential returning nurse.
- to provide work experience in a secure setting with super-vision.

Although the hospital authority is hoping to recruit new staff members, joining the back-to-nursing course is not conditional on accepting employment. There is no obligation at the outset of the course for members to commit themselves in any way to future employment. Some authorities may charge a small amount for attendance at the course, often refundable if the nurse does join the staff, as this weeds out the 'interested' people from those seriously considering employment.

Indeed, a back-to-nursing course can be a testing ground for a woman to see if she might like to return to work and to assess how a job would fit into her family life. Or the course could be a jumping-off point, whereby she might gain sufficient confidence to seek a job in an allied field, such as in a general practitioner surgery or old people's home.

Organisation of the course

As there is no standard course to which we can refer, the accompanying timetable in Figure 4.1 is a proposed back-to-nursing

		Monday	Tuesday	Wednesday	Thursday
	9.30 am to	Introduction to course plan and members	Structure of NHS and nursing management hierarchy	SI units	*DNE* UKCC. Training programmes and assessment Basic and continuing courses
	10.30 am		COFFEE		
W E E K	11 am to	Local district health facilities and tour of hospital	Aseptic technique Classroom demonstration and practice with dressing packs	Drug legislation and administration Simulated drug round and use of charts	*Practical revision* Revise urinalysis, injections and blood pressure
1	12.30 pm		LUNCH		
	1.15 pm	The nursing process and planned nursing care	*Visit* CSSD Cross infection control	Revise pre- and post-op care as group work	*Ward of choice* Observe and shadow a trained nurse
	2 pm	*Visit* Geriatric unit Admission procedure and nursing history	*Visit* Surgical unit Demonstration of removal of sutures	*Visit* Theatre and recovery ward	
	3 pm	using Kardex			

	M	T	W	T
9.30 am to	*District administrator* Legal aspects of nursing	*RCN Rep* Role of the RCN	*Group work* management Exercise in problem solving	*Finance officer* Salaries, superannuation, insurance and tax
10.30 am	COFFEE			
11 am to	*Practical revision* Intravenous infusion and additives Blood transfusion Catheterisation	Cardiopulmonary resuscitation The crash call trolley *Film* Crash call	Fire lecture Evacuation drill and use of extinguisher *Film* Hospitals Don't Burn Down	*Ward of choice* Observe and shadow a trained nurse
12.30 pm	LUNCH			
1.15 pm	*Visit* A & E and OPD	*Visit* ITU and CCU	*Visit* Paediatric unit	*DNO* Career opportunities Bank nursing Board courses Part-time work
2 pm	Revision of first aid and bandaging	*Physiotherapist* Lifting and using hoists	*Social worker* Community links and facilities	*Discussion* Evaluation of course
3 pm	*Film* Don't Let Him Die			

WEEK 2

Fig. 4.1   A proposed plan for a back-to-nursing course.

course, a composite devised from some that have been success-fully used, together with suggestions by returning nurses.

Because it is so common for women to make the decision to pursue a return to work when their children are at full-time school, it is imperative that any course should fit in with school hours and avoid school holiday periods. Daytime courses, organised between 9.30 am and 3 pm, may be arranged for one day a week for six or eight weeks, or twice weekly for a month or run for a full week or fortnight.

Some hospitals may have difficulty fitting a daytime course in with their busy training schedule, so may organise a weekly evening class, similar to local authority evening class sessions. As this may incur expenses for hire of a hall or college of further education, as well as fees for lecturers, course members may be charged a small sum to attend, comparable with evening class fees.

The most likely arrangement is for day courses to be held in the nurses' training school, organised by the teaching staff and making use of the clinical situations at suitable times. A nominal sum may be asked to cover the expense of photocopied handouts and the hire of special films, but, in general, the cost is borne by the hospital, making use of staff in their employ and school premises and equipment.

Course organisers who have tried to make a back-to-nursing course a self-financing venture without burden to the health authority have found nurses very willing to pay a reasonable amount for the opportunity of updating their professional knowledge.

One reasonable option, as shown in the timetable, is to plan a course lasting for two weeks, running for three or four days each week. This gives course members a day or two free to catch up with domestic chores and does allow a gentler introduction to the work-type situation. It gives families an idea of how they might be able to accommodate to a working mother, and for the woman to see how she can adjust to fitting together a job and running the home.

Also to be considered is that course members are plunged into an exacting situation, in immediate contrast to their homely lifestyle. They can expect to feel thoroughly exhausted by the whole mental, physical, emotional and social experience, despite the fact that everything is so interesting and stimulating!

Mealbreaks of coffee and lunch can be taken in the hospital canteen, to be paid for by course members, or packed lunch can be brought in. These informal refreshment breaks are an invaluable time for members to develop into a cohesive group, to unwind and evaluate their feelings and reactions to what they are seeing. In general discussion, they can air problems and are able to identify similar anxieties amongst colleagues. No one is alone in feeling foolish about worrying over a certain aspect of their work or fumbling with practical gadgets. Tutors are also well placed to assess the progress of the course and identify any special areas of need.

Course structure

The core content of any course will be broadly similar to the topics included within this book, with the added bonus of the practical situation. Being on hospital premises enables members to soak up the environment and to mingle with hospital staff, who can impart their special expertise in their clinical area. Nurses can ask immediate queries at the grass roots level, whenever they arise. Being involved in a group, the women are cushioned from feelings of isolation and inadequacy, by sharing the ups and downs of other members, similarly placed, with similar misgivings, fears and doubts.

It is beneficial that potential nurses become acquainted with a variety of colleagues from all aspects of hospital life, which forms an important part of the orientation process. Wherever possible, the organising tutor will invite staff members to talk about their particular field of responsibility. The district fire officer can give a lecture on fire hazards and evacuation methods, the administrator is on hand to discuss legal aspects, the director of nursing can talk about training programmes and post-basic opportunities. The finance officer could be recruited to discuss matters of pay and employment, and the social worker and the dietician on site could offer their services along with many other specialists.

Ward and department staff will be met in their clinical situation, to take the group on a conducted tour and point out matters of interest in that area. The physiotherapist could demonstrate lifting techniques and the use of hoists in her department, while the intensive care unit sister could talk about her role and demonstrate equipment in her unit, in particular the cardiac arrest trolley and its contents. Being shown around a clinical area is worth a hundred lectures on the same subject, and it is a part of the course which returning nurses find most valuable to them.

Of course the supreme advantage of a hospital-based back-to-nursing course is in being able to give members the opportunity to handle equipment and charts and practise techniques in the 'safety' of the classroom, before approaching real patients. Wherever possible, it is advisable for practical procedures to be demonstrated in the authentic clinical environment, for example to see sutures removed from a real patient. However, it is of the utmost value to allow the returning nurse ample opportunity to reinforce her skills by getting plenty of practice in the training school.

A back-to-nursing course is an updating course and there is a limit to how much revision of theory can be incorporated in a short time. The nurse will be expected to be conversant with basic anatomy and physiology and may be asked to read around certain subjects prior to the course, especially concerning the cardiovascular, respiratory and urinary systems.

It is always educationally beneficial to match theory with related practice. So the theoretical sessions on SI units and drug legislation, for example, would be followed by a simulated drug round with the charts in current use. A demonstration and practice of cardiopulmonary resuscitation, would be reinforced with a film and followed by a visit to an intensive care unit to talk about the cardiac arrest procedure. An aseptic technique can be practised in the classroom and demonstrated on a ward, together with a visit to the central sterile supply department (CSSD) to hear about cross-infection control and see how sterile packs are prepared.

With a lot of new information to absorb, it is important to punctuate theory with stimulating speakers, films, demonstrations and visits. A school of nursing will have a good stock of visual aid material and library books, which can be used to good advantage in a back-to-nursing course.

As a rule of thumb, 'heavy' theoretical subjects are best tackled early in the day, while everyone is fresh, alert and attentive. Practical sessions, visits and discussions can be kept until later in the day, when members are flagging—notably after lunch, with the notorious postprandial lag!

A course should be structured to give occasions where members can pool their ideas on a project. An example would be to revise the preoperative and postoperative care regime or work out a situational problem in a management exercise. This all helps to get the group gelled together, and allows individuals to see just how much they can remember and to realise that they have more to offer than they may have originally thought. Groups of mature people are not usually reticent with project work or talking to visiting speakers and are well able to contribute to discussions and ask whatever they feel they need to know.

It would be impossible to endeavour to include everything that all nurses might encounter back at work, considering the diversity of clinical areas to which each might be allocated.

The aim is to provide a broad-based introduction to general topics of relevance to the modern nurse and update aspects which will be vital to any nurse in any field of employment. This should give her a firm basis from which to start, to stimulate thoughts and instil interest for her personal continued study. Any back-to-nursing course would include crucial items on current organisation, practice and methods, such as cardiopulmonary resuscitation (CPR), metric calculations, drug legislation, fire and safety, changes in NHS organisation and nurses' statutory bodies, the nursing process and practical revision of blood pressure recording, injections, intravenous infusions and aseptic technique.

Local variations in course content would depend on the specialty care given in any particular hospital and the type of work likely to confront the returning nurse. In a cancer hospital there would be emphasis on pain control, care of the dying and handling of cytotoxic drugs. A nurse working in a chest hospital would need added instruction on management of underwater seal drainage, removal of chest drains and revision on thoracentesis. In an orthopaedic situation the nurse would need to be conversant with traction and plaster of Paris.

Nurses on a back-to-nursing course invariably think they would like the course to be longer, and this is a reflection of the interest generated in their work. But there is a limit to the amount of teaching that is useful and you soon enter the realms of diminishing returns. Any extra time is more profitably spent gaining additional periods of real ward experience, with on-the-job instruction suited to the aspects of care special to that area.

Work experience

The resounding cry from the returning nurse is for more time allocated to the wards, more supervised practice and more guidance in those initial few weeks at work.

Hospitals will vary in the way that they choose to ease nurses back to the working environment and to their safe and confident role of responsibility. Obviously it is helpful if the nurse has spent a good deal of course time in and around the wards and departments. Nurses are able to gauge the kind of environment, and to some extent the kind of people, with whom they might like to work. A perceptive sister who shows a welcoming, encouraging attitude to a group of visiting returning nurses, may be gratified by new staff keen to work alongside her.

If the staff situation is good, the returning nurse may be put on the ward roster as a supernumary staff nurse, to shadow the regular trained nurse. She will not be left in charge initially, until both she and the nursing officer feel she is fully competent to assume complete responsibility. During this time, it is useful if the clinical instructor can take the new nurse under her wing, to give extra tuition and instructional sessions relevant to that area of work.

Alternatively, the nurse may be assigned to a less technical area, such as the outpatient department, geriatrics or continuing care, where she can function well and develop her role. Or the nurse may choose to join the nurse bank to take on relief duties.

Sometimes, a nurse will complete the course and still remain unsure whether she can commit herself to a job or if she feels confident to return to nursing. In this situation, she may be assigned to a ward, in an unpaid volunteer capacity, wearing a white coat, to shadow and observe the trained nurses and help with basic duties. She cannot assume the responsibilities of a qualified nurse, as she is not legally covered by being employed by the authority but will benefit from a longer ward experience.

Whichever way the hospital decides to employ the returning nurse after completion of the course, each nurse must feel assured that she has the full support of the trained staff and can approach the nursing officer with any problems. It is also useful if she can be informally assigned to a member of the teaching staff, to whom she may refer for advice and guidance, providing a good link between the training school and the service side.

Conclusion

It is difficult for hospitals to predict the positive outcome of a back-to-nursing course, as members often join with ill-defined ideas about their prospects of future employment. If a course is widely advertised, there is invariably an enormous response from interested nurses, many who make the effort to attend and always find the experience most worthwhile.

A lot of members are placed in a part-time position, while others find that the nurse bank is an appealing way to work on an occasional basis, with the prospect of permanent work later on.

Some members do realise at that particular time, that it would be impossible for them to reconcile the demands of both family and job. Family circumstances do dictate the ability of working women to offer themselves for employment. However, from a public relations point of view, the course has offered a favourable introduction to the hospital and local services, which may encourage those nurses to seek work in the near future.

In general, it would seem that hospitals offering a comprehensive back-to-nursing course, backed up by a substantial period of supervised practice which is sympathetic to the needs of the returning nurse, fare better in gaining and retaining happy and proficient new nurses. Nothing could be more terrifying than a cursory introduction, followed by being thrown into the deep end and left to flounder.

Induction/orientation course

It is advisable that every employee, in any type of business, spends a reasonable amount of time getting acquainted with the new environment and learning about local policies and work practices. This introductory period may be called induction or orientation, and is required to ease staff safely and happily into their new place of work.

Large hospitals which have groups of people frequently joining the staff, may run a multidisciplinary induction course at regular intervals, to embrace all new staff in a wide range of occupations: porters, chefs, cleaners, physiotherapists, secretaries and nurses. This would be geared to include aspects of the employment scene that are common to all new staff, such as health and safety, fire drill, labour relations, lifting, together with an orientation to departments and personnel.

Alternatively, an induction course specifically designed for new nurses would be arranged to cover policies and procedures directly related to their work which are peculiar to that hospital: for example, cardiac arrest procedure, ordering stocks, pharmacy, diets, booking investigations, report sheets, special checklists, uniform policy, last offices etc. It should also include practical demonstrations and visits to clinical areas, as well as a period of shadowing a trained nurse, to allow the new nurse to gradually assume her role. This type of induction is useful for any nurse joining a new organisation, especially, for example, a nurse changing from an NHS hospital to work in the private sector,

where management and administrative affairs are handled somewhat differently.

Any induction period is only meant as an orientation to a nurse
who is already well versed in current nursing methods, and is not
expected to offer an updating on training. However, an authority
wishing to employ a returning nurse and being sympathetic to
her needs could easily adapt and extend an induction course to
give more instruction and work experience for the woman who
requires more supervised practice.

Refresher course

Some health authorities run refresher courses for trained nurses,
often in response to requests for general post-basic tuition. This
initiative by nurses, and the fact that refresher courses are enthusiastically taken up, is an indication of the interest shown by
qualified nurses, who are obviously keen to further their personal
knowledge of the profession.

Most courses are at present outside the normal educational
structure and are usually organised on an evening class basis,
bringing speakers to offer their specialist expertise. Because they
have to be self-financing courses, a small charge is often made to
cover expenses and lecture fees.

Refresher courses are not intended to update nurses in a retro-
spective direction, as does a back-to-nursing course, so they do
not aim to cater specifically for resting nurses who have been out
of the profession for years. It would largely be presumed that
course members are au fait with current nursing practice, so the
updating is on a more horizontal level, by boosting the fund of
knowledge on a wider basis.

Most practising nurses have their work confined to one area
and may feel that their knowledge is concentrated, and fairly
limited, to that narrow field. A nurse who knows a lot about der-
matology may be interested to know about the work of the
district nurse, to whose care her patients are discharged. The
health visitor might be keen to find out about the latest treatment
regimes used in cancer or to understand more about epidural
anaesthesia and ultrasound, techniques about which her antenatal patients may enquire. A variety of topics are common to
virtually every area of care, like diabetes, arthritis, pressure
sores, pain and dying, and deeper study about any of these would

be beneficial for nurses to improve their understanding and subsequent care of patients.

All nurses would like to be kept abreast of important changes within the health service or nursing practice as and when they occur. So they would welcome a discussion of any new organisational structure of the NHS, to be informed of legal developments, such as the Mental Health Act or the introduction of new methods, like SI units or insulin strengths.

Refresher courses are offered to any qualified nurse who wishes to avail herself of the service. Course members largely comprise those currently employed in nursing, perhaps in the hospital service in a restricted area like a theatre nurse or a phlebotomist; nurses in primary health care such as district nurse, health visitor, school nurse, general practice nurse, as well as occupational health nurses in industry. They are particularly appealing to nurses employed on a part-time basis, who are keen to broaden their scope of information about their profession in this most satisfactory way.

If a refresher course is advertised in the locality, a resting nurse could take advantage of joining and attend in a similar way to an evening class. This could be an ideal way for a nurse to keep abreast of changes within the profession, whether or not she was intending to return to nursing in the near future.

Figure 4.2 outlines a simulated refresher course, which gives an idea of the type of subjects that may be arranged to interest qualified nurses.

Further study

If there are no back-to-nursing or refresher courses available in your locality, there are other ways you can remain informed about the profession and become reacquainted with study.

The most obvious method to keep abreast of changes within the profession is to read the nursing journals on a regular basis. The secret of using these as an effective tool for study is by making a positive intention to read those articles that *do not* immediately capture your interest. Any items that you *choose* to read are likely to be something on which you know a lot about already, while the articles that you feel inclined to gloss over are probably the ones that you need most!

Refresher Course for Qualified Nurses

10 Study Evenings in Nursing School

Time: 7–9.30 pm Fee: £10 per course

Theme	Sessions	Speaker
Modern philosophy of nursing	Nursing models of care Application of nursing process Modern nurse training	Tutor Sister Tutor
Care of the elderly	Team assessment, geriatric unit Preventive care in community Support of elderly mentally infirm	Sister of unit Health visitor Community psychiatric nurse
Pain	Physiology and psychology of pain Pain control in terminal illness Transcutaneous nerve stimulation	Tutor Oncology sister Physiotherapist
Diabetes	Current treatment Management in hospital and home Diabetic diet	Doctor Diabetic liaison sister Dietician
Coronary heart disease	Pathology of CHD. ECG readings Surgical correction Medical and surgical care in ICU	Doctor Doctor ICU sister
Care of the dying patient and the family	Hospice care The patient dying at home Bereavement (discussion)	Hospice sister Macmillan sister Social worker
Bowel surgery	Surgical techniques Specialised nursing care Stoma management in and out of hospital	Doctor Sister Stoma liaison sister
Oncology	Choices in cancer therapy Paediatric oncology The woman with breast cancer	Doctor Paediatric sister Breast care sister
Joint disease	Osteoarthritis, surgical care Rheumatoid arthritis Help to independence	Tutor Sister OT
Contemporary role of the nurse	Health education Accountability A problem-solving exercise	Health educationalist Tutor Tutor
Conclusion	Evaluation of course and ideas for further courses	

Fig. 4.2   *An example of a proposed refresher course for trained nurses.*

Television and radio documentaries and the better Sunday papers are also a good source of up-to-date information on contemporary, and often contentious, medical and social matters of public, and therefore professional, interest.

The British Red Cross Society and the St John Ambulance Association organise courses in first aid, home nursing and, sometimes, mental health care and preventive medicine. Although geared to instruct the public in rudiments of care and emergency assistance, nurses would benefit from involvement in these classes, to stimulate their interest and revise their basic skills, by joining in and contributing with other participants. Indeed, the first aid classes may be very illuminating. For, contrary to popular opinion, nurses are not particularly expert at first aid, as they quickly become reliant on the availability of professional help and equipment at hand, rather than learning how to improvise in an emergency situation beyond the hospital gates.

Any nurse who is free to attend a local authority evening or day class would be well advised to select a subject appropriate to her profession. Modern nurse training programmes include psychology and sociology as applied to health care. So, these behavioural sciences would be useful topics with which to become reacquainted, as would human biology, general biology or chemistry, especially if further study within nursing is anticipated at a later stage. Even without the intention of sitting the final examination, the course of study would be stimulating and informative, while persistence with a class is a good boost for morale.

Some enterprising nurses use their years at home most profitably by gaining a degree, usually through the Open University, which allows people to study at home and is particularly useful for mothers confined with young children. Taking Open University courses involves considerable expense and is certainly only to be recommended to the most highly motivated people, who could be enthusiastic and diligent students able to commit themselves to sustained study over a number of years.

However, the Open University programmes broadcast on TV are freely available for anyone to view and much of the material has relevance to nurses.

A special Open University package has been designed for nurses called, 'A systematic approach to nursing care' (see page 208). Although it is available for individuals to study at home, it is meant to provide the core material for tutors to use in group work, where there is access to clinical experience.

The resting nurse may be interested to read around those subjects applicable to the Diploma in Nursing, in preparation for future study. It is a three-year course on a part-time basis, under the auspices of the extramural department of the University of London, aimed at advanced study of nursing (see page 202). Depending on her background experience and education, the nurse could enrol for the first year of the Diploma in Nursing course at a college, although this would incur substantial fees and does require attendance for one full day every week.

For the second and third years, the nurse would have to be in a clinical placement, in substantial part-time or full-time work, as these parts of the course involve care planning and clinical application of the theory.

Any nurse interested in finding out about the Dip N should inquire at the extramural department for preliminary details and then at the local college which operates the course.

Of course *any* form of recent relevant study would be impressive to an employer, demonstrating interest and motivation in the prospective nurse employee.

New opportunities for women (NOW courses)

Some local colleges offer courses to mature students and details of these can be found in the library.

Certain courses are geared to help adults who may either have missed out on formal education in earlier years or those who have not seen the inside of a classroom for a long time and wish to brush up their academic skills. The latter would apply to many nurses who, having completed their basic nurse training many years ago, have not applied themselves to serious study since that time.

Other courses are intended to reorientate mature women to the work scene, for those who have been absent from outside employment for a number of years and are feeling diffident about offering themselves for work. Women are encouraged to take stock of their abilities and attributes, with advice on jobseeking, the completion of a curriculum vitae or application forms, interviewing technique, together with counselling on career prospects.

These types of courses bear the title of something akin to 'Fresh

Start', 'New Horizons' or 'Back to Work' and give very positive advice. Although not specifically orientated towards nursing, such a course may provide a useful opportunity for nurses to meet like-minded women, and be helped to explore their potential, sharpen communication skills and boost their confidence.

Reference and refresher reading

Cox, C. (1983). *Sociology: Introduction for Nurses, Midwives and Health Visitors*. London: Butterworths.

Hall, J. (1982). *Psychology for Nurses and Health Visitors*. London: Macmillan.

5

Organisational Structures

The National Health Service

At the inception of the NHS in 1948, the original tripartite structure of organisation delivered health care from three distinctly separate sources.

The hospital services were administered by the management committees of regional hospital boards and by the boards of governors of teaching hospitals. Community services, comprising the health centre, district nursing, community midwifery, health visiting, ambulance service and preventive health care, were the responsibility of the local authority health department. Executive councils arranged the general practitioner, dental, ophthalmic and pharmaceutical services.

However this disunited approach did little for smooth liaison or continuity of patient care, with one of two results. A patient might have received multiple, repetitious help from several sources, or slip through the net of communication and receive none.

The major reorganisation of the NHS in 1974 was aimed at unification of the service, to provide integrated health care and manage funding more efficiently. This comprehensive health system was rearranged as a three-tier structure, dividing the United Kingdom into regional health authorities (RHA), each of which was further divided into area health authorities (AHA). Most of the AHAs were further organised into districts on a geographical basis, the units which were to actually administer health care to people at the grass roots.

It soon became evident that the middle tier was superfluous to operational needs. The area level was a monstrous waste of valuable NHS money and manpower, hindering quick and effective decision-making both up and down the hierarchy of power.

So in 1982, in an effort to reduce the bureaucracy and increase efficiency within the service, the NHS was subjected to another minor shuffle, in which the AHAs were abandoned. Their functions were absorbed by newly formed and named district health authorities (DHA), who related directly to their RHA.

The current structure can be succinctly summed up by saying that health care planning, involving decisions of priorities and allocation of expenditure occurs centrally, whereas its implementation occurs locally (see Figure 5.1).

The Department of Health and Social Security (DHSS)

The DHSS, headed by the Secretary of State for Social Services, has the national responsibility for (1) the NHS, (2) social services, and (3) social security. All of these are financed from the Exchequer, paid for largely by general taxation and National Insurance contributions.

The DHSS plans for future health care provision, taking account of demography—projected changes in population; and epidemiology—the manifestation of health trends and their geographical distribution. It needs to anticipate and be equipped to cope with future developments, such as the increase in the elderly population, the transition of the handicapped into the community, control of drug abuse. It is also necessary to spread out the specialist facilities, rather than concentrating everything in cities and teaching hospitals. For example, every region would be asked to ensure that there are reasonable facilities for neonatal intensive care and renal dialysis, rather than have patients around the country in search of adequate treatment.

As the master planner, with the hold on the pursestrings, the DHSS has to decide how to distribute its limited resources for the maximum benefit of the population as a whole. The government is quite sensitive to requests made by pressure groups, who have the interest of any particular group to serve, be they professional workers or the public, such as the Child Poverty Action Group or Action on Smoking and Health (ASH).

Regional health authorities

In England, there are 14 regional health authorities responsible for between 8 and 22 DHAs. They allocate resources to their constituent districts, plan the development of health needs forecast within the geographical area which they serve, and schedule capital developments. RHAs also coordinate research projects and training programmes, employ senior professional staff and maintain a blood transfusion service. Each RHA has within its

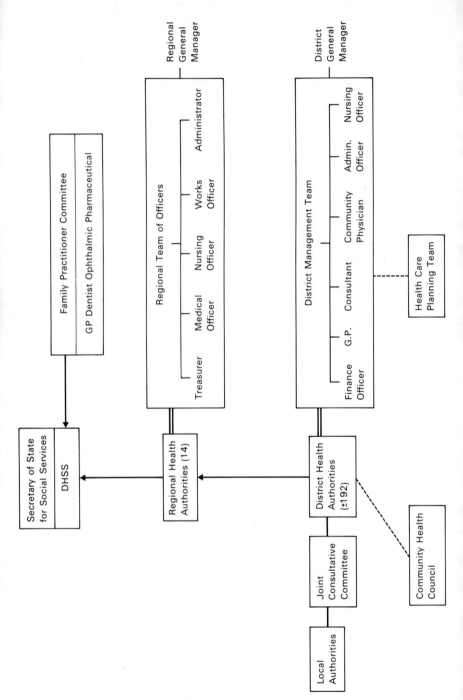

Fig. 5.1   A simplified framework of the NHS structure.

boundary at least one university providing medical education.

An RHA is served by five officers, forming the regional team of officers (RTO), comprising a doctor, nurse, works officer, administrator and treasurer, who collectively recommend regional forward planning policies and also monitor the performance of DHAs.

District health authorities

The district health authorities, 192 in England, are accountable to their RHA. A DHA is the basic unit of day-to-day management and delivery of health care to the nation at local level. It provides the full range of care for local needs, both in hospital and in the community, which may vary from place to place and from time to time, to reflect the predominant requirements, whether it be a population with a lot of elderly or handicapped or one with young families or an area with high unemployment or a transient population to cater for.

District services may be an amalgam of smaller units of older hospitals, brought under one umbrella designation. But, a new district general hospital (DGH) should incorporate all the required specialist hospital services, and rationalise the use of the paramedical and ancillary facilities.

District management team
A district management team (DMT) serves the DHA to manage the services within the district, to coordinate hospital and community amenities, and to plan and evaluate performance within their district. The DMT comprises the district community physician, district nursing officer, district administrator, district finance officer, plus a general practitioner and consultant who act as chairman and vice-chairman.

Until recently, the DMT held the responsibility to make policy decisions by consensus agreement. The *Griffiths report* on management in the NHS forms the latest reappraisal of the system and has led to the appointment of general managers at regional and district level.

District general manager
Each district has a district general manager (DGM) appointed by members of the DHA and approved by the Minister, initially

for a three-year fixed-term contract. Anyone with a proven managerial ability is eligible to become a general manager. Some have been derived from the original DMT and have a professional background, either doctors or nurses, a treasurer or administrator. Yet many others have been sought from outside the health service, whose previous experience has been in management within commercial organisations.

The DGM will have the ultimate responsibility to deploy the limited resources that are available for a district to the maximum benefit of the population. A business style of management is being applied to the NHS to provide cost-effective functioning of the service, with an overall philosophy aimed at 'getting things done', by avoiding a cumbersome bureaucratic machinery and relating to one individual in charge.

Obviously, the DGM will need to liaise with the specialist officers of the DMT and rely on their expertise, in order to gain an overall perspective of the disciplines. This is a prerequisite to ensure that policies are formulated for the effective and efficient delivery of health care. But the role of the general manager is a new one and there is no way of predicting how each DGM may decide to arrange the managerial responsibility within each health authority. This may result in still more restructuring of the NHS in the future.

Health care planning teams

Health care planning teams are made up of staff from a wide range of disciplines, working together to assess and recommend for the ongoing and anticipated needs in the district.

Joint consultative committees

Joint consultative committees are a combination of health care staff and local authority staff who meet to advise on the organisation of the health, social and educational services, which overlap to serve the population.

Community health council

To improve accountability to the consumer, each district has a community health council (CHC) appointed to represent the interest of the residents in the local community. It provides an opportunity for local people to have a say in the development of health services within their community and allows for a feedback on performance of the service and satisfaction of the patient.

Family practitioner committee

The family practitioner committee is responsible for all general practitioner, dental, optical and pharmaceutical services and it relates directly to the DHSS.

The health service commissioners for England and Wales

The health service commissioners for England and Wales are available to make independent enquiries into complaints against any of the health bodies within the NHS and are used by people who feel they have had dissatisfaction from the service.

All that has been said about the organisation of the NHS has been relevant to England only, and there are variations in administration in other parts of the United Kingdom.

Local authority social services

Prior to 1970, social workers employed by the local authority had a specific responsibility to groups of clients with similar needs, specialising either in the handicapped, the blind, the elderly, children or mental welfare. The medical social worker (MSW) and psychiatric social worker (PSW) were employed directly by the hospital authority.

Reorganisation, upon recommendation by the Seebohm report (1968), resulted in a generic social work department in the local authority, with MSW and PSW under their jurisdiction. All social workers now assume a generic role, which equips them to deal with all aspects of need within one family, whereas before several social workers may have overlapped in caring for individuals in one family—one for the handicapped child, another for the depressed mother and another for the old granny all within the same household.

The Central Council for Education and Training in Social Work has the responsibility of maintaining standards of training within social work. A basic two-year course leads to the Certificate of Qualification in Social Work (CQSW); candidates with a degree in social sciences may take a shortened course. There are also training courses for social work assistants or aids, who largely help out with the practical aspects of the work.

Social workers based in hospitals are allocated from the social services department of the local authority and form an essential part of the health care team. They have a major role in counselling, while also having at their fingertips an immense knowledge of the resources, with amenities, personnel and benefits, which can best serve the patient and his family, both in hospital and on discharge.

There are obvious benefits in forging links between health and social workers and their departments. Their work frequently overlaps and coincides, in hospital and now with the increasing emphasis of care in the community. The administration of the DHAs are coterminous with the local authority and the school and housing authorities, which means they function within the same geographical boundary.

Nursing staff structure

The nursing profession has been involved in a battery of changes over the last 20 years, some directly concerning its own staff structure and responsibility, others indirectly as a result of reorganisations in the health service generally. It is important to realise that with each turbulent upheaval, many senior, experienced nurses leave the profession prematurely, rather than join a gruelling jostle for jobs and be subjected to arduous and unsettling rearrangement of their lives. It may all be in the cause of progress but frequent disturbance of order takes its toll on the service and on individuals.

'Management' has been the key word responsible for the many changes, in an effort to get it right for an efficient health service.

The first major reorganisation for the profession began in 1966, with the start of the implementation of the Salmon structure for senior nursing staff. Matron and her assistants, who administered from a central location, were rejected in favour of a hierarchy of nursing management, based on clinical areas of responsibility. New titles and grades, numbering from 5 to 10, indicated the level of managerial responsibility. It introduced the concept of the nursing officer, responsible for a group of clinical departments, who in turn was accountable to a senior nursing officer, with a wider area of supervision. These grades are used less specifically now and may be replaced by senior nurse or clinical unit manager.

Changes within the NHS have by necessity modified the Salmon structure, particularly at the more senior levels, with an alteration in titles, but the basic administrative idea of line management in a hierarchy still exists.

All nursing staff are employed by the DHA, whether they work in hospital or the community, and this obviously fosters good liaison between these two major areas of care.

As shown on the left-hand side of Figure 5.2, the district nursing officer (DNO), a member of the DMT, is the head of all nursing services within that district. Each major division is supervised by a director, so there is a director of nursing service (DNS) for the general division, psychiatry (including mental handicap), midwifery (including domiciliary midwifery), community and primary care services, and a director of nurse education (DNE) for the training division. Some of these larger areas of responsibility may also command an assistant director post.

Within each of these divisions is a hierarchy of management down to ward level and up again, as demonstrated in the right-hand side of Figure 5.2, with the general division in detail.

A senior nurse will take responsibility for a specified area, such as night duty or a combination of accident and emergency, outpatients departments, theatres, or a small local hospital. Within that clinical unit are several wards or departments, each managed by a sister or charge nurse.

Some nurses do not fit into this line structure, as they are individual practitioners whose work may cover the whole of a hospital or district, such as nurses working in personnel, occupational health, counselling, patient care development or staff in-service training.

The statutory bodies for nursing, midwifery and health visiting

The General Nursing Council (GNC) no longer exists as the statutory body responsible for the training and registration of nurses. Gone also are the Central Midwives Board (CMB), the

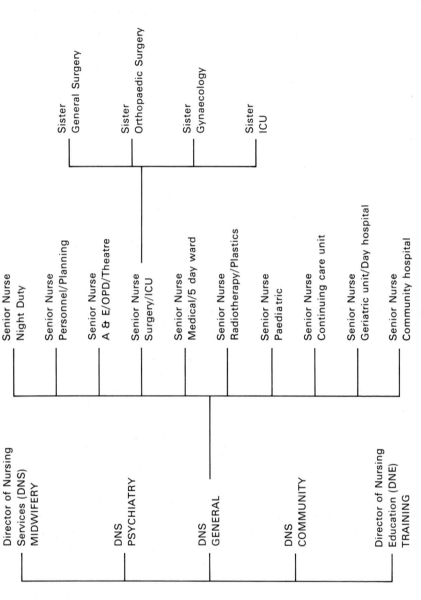

Fig. 5.2   An example of the senior nursing staff structure within a district.

Council for the Education and Training of Health Visitors (CETHV), the Panel of Assessors for District Nurse Training (PADNT), the Joint Board of Clinical Nursing Studies (JBCNS) and their equivalent bodies in Scotland and Northern Ireland.

The UKCC

In 1983, altogether nine statutory bodies responsible for all nursing, midwifery and health visiting in the United Kingdom were discontinued. Their responsibilities were amalgamated under the umbrella administration of the United Kingdom Central Council (UKCC) and *four national boards*: English National Board (ENB), Welsh National Board (WNB), National Board for Scotland (NBS), National Board for Northern Ireland (NBNI). The five bodies function coexistently and interdependently, having the shared responsibility for the training, education and maintenance of all nurses, midwives and health visitors in the United Kingdom (see Figure 5.3).

The UKCC holds the central register of qualified staff. It also formulates central policies as regards training and standards, which the national boards implement and supervise at local level. This includes the training syllabuses and assessments, together with approval of training establishments and their courses.

The Briggs Report

This momentous change was initiated by a proposal from the Report by the Committee on Nursing (the Briggs Report, 1970), as a result of this exhaustive evaluation of the structure of nursing service and education. The basic recommendation was for a unified structure that would provide more rational and effective patterns of training and delivery of care. The suggestion was not unanimously applauded from all parts of the profession, especially those branches of nursing with smaller numbers, who felt that their interests might be overshadowed by those with a greater representation.

However, this proposal from the Briggs Report did reach the statute book, to become law in 1979, as the Nurses, Midwives and Health Visitors Act.

Other proposals regarding training and continuing education

Previous Bodies

GNC
GNCS
CMB
CMBS
CETHV
CCNS
PADNT
NICNM
JBCNS

New Bodies

U	ENB
K	WNB
C	NBS
C	NBNI

Combined Responsibilities

Registration

Training

Education

Professional standards

Professional conduct

Investigations of misconduct
and unfitness to practise

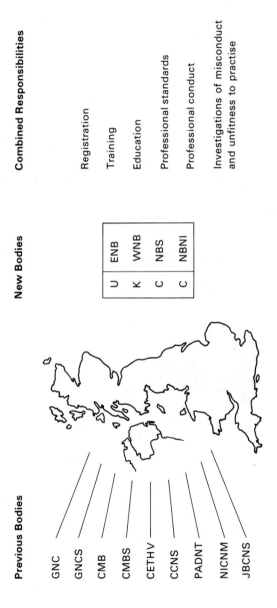

Fig. 5.3 The reorganisation of the statutory bodies for nursing, midwifery and health visiting in the UK. Nine statutory bodies were combined into five new ones.

are being considered by the newly formed bodies and may result in a major reorganisation of nurse training as we know it. Current systems of training for registration and enrolment will continue until such time as the new bodies advise otherwise.

The previous JBCNS courses are now called post-basic clinical courses, under the direction of their relevant national body and referred to by numbers, for example ENB no. 264—course in Burns and Plastic Surgery Nursing for Registered General Nurses.

The Joint Examination Board which used to be responsible for orthopaedic nurse training has also ceased to function. Clinical courses will be available for the post-basic orthopaedic specialty but there is no longer any provision for 17-year-old nurses to do it as a pre-basic course prior to general training.

All five bodies—the UKCC and the four national boards—have responsibilities towards professional conduct, which is obviously concerned with safety of the vulnerable public in the hands of competent practitioners (see Figure 5.4). They hold enquiries into allegations of misconduct and the Council is empowered to remove names from the register, which may be restored at a later date. One new mechanism is a Health Committee, which investigates alleged cases of 'unfitness to practice due to mental or physical ill health', if a practitioner seems medically unfit to work, either temporarily or permanently. It removes the traumatic, disciplinary attitude and replaces it with one that is sensitive, caring and helping, and often provides the first step towards professional rehabilitation.

The Briggs Report also recommended very strongly that nursing should become a research-based profession. The UKCC has a Research Committee to initiate and facilitate research and to advise the Council on matters relating to research in nursing.

SPRINT

The initial major task for the UKCC was to compile and maintain a single professional register, from the diverse records of the disbanded bodies. Information about all trained nurses, midwives and health visitors is stored on a central computer.

This new register is known as SPRINT-UK (Single Professional Register–Index of Training–UK). A single entry for each individual records that person's relevant details from the

Each registered nurse, midwife and health visitor shall act, at all times, in such a manner as to justify public trust and confidence, to uphold and enhance the good standing and reputation of the profession, to serve the interests of society, and above all to safeguard the interests of individual patients and clients.

Each registered nurse, midwife and health visitor is accountable for his or her practice, and in the exercise of professional accountability shall:

1 Act always in such a way as to promote and safeguard the wellbeing and interests of patients/clients.

2 Ensure that no action or omission on his/her part or within his/her sphere of influence is detrimental to the condition or safety of patients/clients.

3 Take every reasonable opportunity to maintain and improve professional knowledge and competence.

4 Acknowledge any limitations of competence and refuse in such cases to accept delegated functions without first having received instruction in regard to those functions and having been assessed as competent.

5 Work in a collaborative and cooperative manner with other health care professionals and recognise and respect their particular contributions within the health care team.

6 Take account of the customs, values and spiritual beliefs of patients/clients.

7 Make known to an appropriate person or authority any conscientious objection which may be relevant to professional practice.

Fig. 5.4   UKCC Code of Professional Conduct for the Nurse, Midwife and Health Visitor.

8 Avoid any abuse of the privileged relationship which exists with patients/clients and of the privileged access allowed to their property, residence or workplace.

9 Respect confidential information obtained in the course of professional practice and refrain from disclosing such information without the consent of the patient/client, or a person entitled to act on his/her behalf, except where disclosure is required by law or by the order of a court or is necessary in the public interest.

10 Have regard to the environment of care and its physical, psychological and social effects on patients/clients, and also to the adequacy of resources, and make known to appropriate persons or authorities any circumstances which could place patient/clients in jeopardy or which militate against safe standards of practice.

11 Have regard to the workload of and the pressures on professional colleagues and subordinates and take appropriate action if these are seen to be such as to constitute abuse of the individual practitioner and/or to jeopardise safe standards of practice.

12 In the context of the individual's own knowledge, experience, and sphere of authority, assist peers and subordinates to develop professional competence in accordance with their needs.

13 Refuse to accept any gift, favour or hospitality which might be interpreted as seeking to exert undue influence to obtain preferential consideration.

14 Avoid the use of professional qualifications in the promotion of commercial products in order not to compromise the independence of professional judgement on which patients/clients rely.

date of entry into training, together with subsequent qualifications.

New standardised titles for each part of the register were introduced, although some do remain the same as before. There is no longer a 'state' badge issued by the registering body for nurses qualifying under the new system. Nurses who attained their qualification prior to 1983 are permitted to continue using those original titles if they so choose (Table 5.1).

Table 5.1 New standardised titles

Part	Designation	Abbrev.	Absorbing
1	For Registered General Nurse	RGN	Previous SRN/RGN
2	For Enrolled Nurses (General)	EN(G)	Previous SEN (England and Wales)
3	For Registered Mental Nurses	RMN	Previous RMN
4	For Enrolled Nurses (Mental)	EN(M)	Previous SEN(M)
5	For Registered Nurses for the Mentally Handicapped	RNMH	Previous RNMS/ RNMD
6	For Enrolled Nurses (Mental Handicap)	EN(MH)	Previous SEN(MS)
7	For Enrolled Nurses	EN	Previous EN, Scotland and SEN, Northern Ireland
8	For Registered Sick Children's Nurses	RSCN	Previous RSCN
9	For Registered Fever Nurses (no longer open to new admissions)	RFN	Previous RFN
10	For Registered Midwives	RM	Previous SCM
11	For Registered Health Visitors	RHV	Previous HV

All nurses who had previously been on one of the old registers or rolls would automatically have been included on SPRINT. However, at present, the UKCC register is not a 'live' register. It merely stores information about *every* nurse who has ever obtained a statutory qualification. Names are only allowed to be removed after official notification has been received to record the death of a nurse.

So, from that list of names there has been no way of checking how many nurses are actually in employment using their qualification, how many are having a rest period or how many have retired. When the register was first compiled, it contained the names of 28 000 nurses over the age of 106! A vast number must also be beyond the age of retirement, while others may have left the profession altogether.

To ensure that the register is a live one, the UKCC is proposing to introduce periodic licensing from January 1987. Every practitioner currently using her qualification will be expected to pay a fee every three years, in order to retain her name on the register, similar to the practice in Scotland. In effect, it will be a licence to practise and will be the responsibility of each nurse and each employer to make sure that the employee is within the law.

This method also enables the UKCC to exercise some control over updating and refreshment of its professionals, similar to the mandatory requirements for midwives. It is hoped that by 1990, some form of compulsory periodic updating will apply, both for nurses in current practice and for the nurse returning after an absence who wish to rejoin the register. As yet, it is unsure precisely what form this periodic refreshment is likely to take, how it will be organised and by whom, or that vital question of who will pay the bill.

By charging practitioners to remain on the register, the UKCC hopes to be funded by its members, thus making it financially independent from government.

In a vast nationwide campaign, the UKCC will attempt to contact all qualified nurses, to get an up-to-date profile of all of those currently in employment. Those who are working will be initiated into periodic licensing and pay the fee which will legally enable them to work for the next three years. Those who are not working will be informed of the requirement to relicense before commencing work.

Some nurses, midwives or health visitors may have missed the publicity regarding these new changes in professional standing, perhaps because they have been abroad, have been untraceable after moving or failed to notice the advertisements.

After January 1987 the nurse seeking a job will be asked to contact the UKCC, get her qualification validated, get relicensed and pay the appropriate fee. This is likely to be between £15 and £20 for a three-year licensing period, payable in total, whether for full-time or part-time work, but is a tax-deductible expense. After 1990, we can presume that the nurse would also be expected to prove that she has been updated and, hopefully, hospitals or colleges will provide recognised courses for returning nurses.

The 1979 Act empowers the new statutory bodies to improve standards of training and professional conduct, which has far-reaching implications for nursing. Although still in their infancy, the new bodies are busily planning for the future development of the nursing profession. This profound challenge provides an exciting time for nurses to re-evaluate their role and function in view of the future health care needs of this nation.

Reference and refresher reading

Davies B. M. (1984). *Community Health and Social Services.* Sevenoaks: Hodder & Stoughton.

6

The Health of the Nation

Changing needs for care

There is no way that the health care planners who organised the NHS in postwar Britain could have envisaged the immense social, economic and technological changes which have affected the nation's health less than half a century later. It is doubtful that they could see much beyond the immediacy of the burning health issues of the day, centred on communicable diseases, control of infection and improvements in standards to provide safer maternity care and give infants a better start in life.

Yet as these menaces were checked and conditions were improved, different problems arose or became manifest, adding to the demands of the health services, such as a higher incidence of coronary heart disease, stress-related disorders, hepatitis, the socially related disorders of alcohol abuse, drug addiction and depression, and the newer frightening epidemics such as AIDS and Legionnaire's disease.

The naive dream of a finite task to clear the United Kingdom of infectious scourges, thereby getting the nation fit and back on its feet, did not materialise. As medicine offered more in the way of health care, then more was demanded, and came to be expected as a right of tax-paying citizens who wanted replacement parts, extended life, a better existence, and new life created in test tubes.

The ideology of the welfare state remains unaltered, and largely unchallenged, although its administration and unwieldy bureaucracy are constantly under scrutiny. Management of health and social services are the responsibility of central government; it is to be free at the point of use and available to all citizens, irrespective of financial status, thereby making equality of entitlement.

Yet the welfare state, like anything which is given freely, finds that it has the potential to generate infinite demands, while having to work with finite resources. This must inevitably result in some rationing and certainly requires sensible allocation of the limited funds.

Health care policies very quickly merge with the contentious areas of politics, economics and ethics. Who has access to the expensive technology? Who is the most 'deserving case'? How can money be put to the most efficient use?

If you take £10 000, for example, it could give one middle-aged man a coronary bypass operation, thereby keeping him in gainful employment in the long-term and his family provided for without recourse to state assistance.

Alternatively, it could pay for ten hip replacements on elderly people, to keep them mobile, active and independent, rather than incurring the cost of continuing care. Or it could be used to renovate a day centre, to give several generations of old people a happier existence near the end of their life.

The same sum could also be directed to a preventive programme for screening a wide population of women, who could be saved from extensive and expensive cancer therapy if their malignancy were detected early.

It could buy two high-tech machines to enable tiny premature babies to grow into normal children. It might be queried whether the same amount of money should be invested in rearing test-tube babies, while another operating theatre is terminating the lives of many healthy, but unwanted, fetuses.

It is all too easy to offer clipped, insensitive financial and political arguments on health facilities, especially when many verge on social engineering. For this avoids the emotional and personal involvement of every issue in human terms, when it might be your precious baby at risk, your mother incapacitated by arthritis or your overwhelming desire to have—or not have—a child.

Several factors may assist in the decisions made for health care planning. One general move is to decentralise specialist facilities, which used to be clustered in the London hospitals and required patients to travel long distances. There are now many more specialist units dotted around the country and Regional authorities instructed to make provisions for a wider range of care, such as dialysis units or leukaemia centres.

The demography of health

Demography is the study of population and, by analysis of changes in sight, forward planning can be organised to match the anticipated need. A baby boom this year will mean an increased

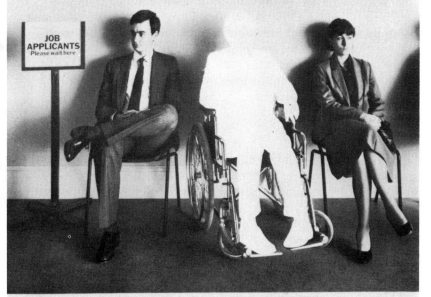

Fig. 6.1 *The importance of changing public attitudes. (Reproduced by kind permission of The Spastics Society.)*

need for paediatric health services and education facilities in the immediate years to come. By projecting these figures further, there will also be a rise in pensioners and concomitant pressure on health services 65 years hence.

Other demographic changes in a society will influence the emergence of patterns of health and disease within that nation of people. We are now witnessing an increase in the elderly within the population, which will continue to rise towards the next century and create a demand for health care.

There is no longer any stigma attached to the single mother bringing up her illegitimate child, and she now joins the ranks of numerous parents who manage alone after divorce or death of a spouse. There is evidence that the unattached suffer from a greater incidence of stress-related diseases than their married colleagues.

Immigrant groups often have special health needs, as do the homeless and jobless. Unemployment, on a scale unimaginable to the population of immediate postwar Britain, brings its own health-related problems, in the form of depression, suicide, family tensions and breakdown and stress-induced illnesses.

Poverty in general has its attendant health and social problems and is spoken of as the 'cycle of deprivation': social demise, poverty and ill-health, a circle from which a person is unable to break free and improve his status.

The law and health

The law plays a significant part in health variations. Witness the Abortion Act in 1967, which put an end to the misery and mortality accompanying illegal abortions, yet put pressure on the NHS gynaecology service to deal with the increased demand for legalised termination of pregnancy, amounting to thousands annually.

A knock-on effect of termination of pregnancy, together with availability of the contraceptive pill, has resulted in a dearth of healthy newborn babies for adoption. The subsequent response has been to stimulate the fervent development of fertility treatments for childless couples who desperately want a child.

The Compulsory Seatbelt Act of 1983 resulted in a dramatic reduction in fatalities and serious injuries, notably of the head and face, of front seat passengers and drivers of vehicles. This law has had a direct effect on the workload of staff in accident and emergency departments and plastic surgery units dealing with faciomaxillary injuries.

Epidemiology

Epidemiology is the study of the incidence of disease affecting a community at a certain time. Knowledge of the distribution of illness can help shape both the curative and preventive health care and social facilities to meet prevailing needs.

It is known that social factors influence the presentation of illness and vary within the different social classes. Class structure is determined by occupation, which in itself is indicative of income level, living conditions, diet, leisure pursuits and social habits.

Despite a general increase in the standard of living, there are still poor families and old people living in a parlous state, whose health is demonstrably worse than their richer neighbours. With less money, less nourishing foods, poorer housing conditions and perhaps less understanding about budgeting and health care, these people continually have a poorer health record. They have a higher level of infant mortality, smaller birthweight of babies, greater incidence of tooth decay in their children, more cancer in their women, and yet show less inclination or knowledge of how to make use of the services available.

There may be some geographical relationship, such as the markedly high incidence of stomach cancer detected in Wales, the greater occurrence of bladder cancer in Scotland or the high incidence of cot deaths and spina bifida in babies born in Milton Keynes. It is worrying also to find an above-average incidence of leukaemias and cancers in the area around a nuclear power station.

Epidemiological variations are also noted between countries, with Japan showing a low incidence of coronary heart disease, compared with Sweden and Scotland, which has the highest in the world. Sweden shows the best record as regards infant mortality, whereas in Europe Portugal has the worst, with the United Kingdom somewhere in between.

Statistics

Epidemiology and demography both rely on the use of statistics, to gather and decipher their evidence. But statistics can only deliver the bare facts of the 'when', 'where' and 'who' of the disease, without being able to conclude the 'why', which requires a lot more investigation to reach the causative factors.

Lung cancer was for a long time a disease most commonly affecting males. Suddenly statistics revealed that it was claiming the lives of many more women, that females were catching up with the figures for the male population. To find out 'why', it was necessary to look at many variables at work, such as the increase in smoking, urban pollution and adoption of more stressful lifestyles.

It is also known that cancer of the breast is more prevalent in women of professional and managerial class than in wives in the unskilled class, yet, curiously, the statistics are totally reversed when considering cancer of the cervix.

Bald statistics in isolation can be very misleading and need to be used guardedly, for it is dangerous to jump to rash conclusions about the meanings behind their interpretation, before further research confirms any hypotheses.

Is there really a greater incidence of heart disease nowadays, or is it that we are screening for it and more aware of its presence? Are there really more cot deaths, or have those unexplained infant deaths in the past been recorded as cases of pneumonia or suffocation?

When statistics show a high infant mortality rate in one area of the country, this only tells you that babies die more frequently there than elsewhere. It might seem obvious to pump in more obstetric and paediatric facilities, only to find that it is an area of economic deprivation and high unemployment, so that pregnant women are poorly nourished, attend antenatal clinics less frequently, and give birth to sickly infants, who start out with a health disadvantage. Despite an overall national improvement in the infant mortality rate, twice as many babies die in the first week of life in social class five, compared to those born into social class one.

It is said that there is a greater incidence of mental illness amongst women. But does this signify that women are more inclined to offer themselves for psychiatric treatment, whereas men keep a stiff upper lip, and women who go to their general practitioner in floods of tears may be labelled and recorded as suffering from depression.

Statistics are an extremely useful tool in this sophisticated age of computerised data collection and analysis, in order to predict patterns of health and to determine future needs, for which we can be adequately prepared in advance. If there are glaring deficiencies in any one area, then suitable aid should be directed to counteract inadequacies in health and social services.

Worldwide health

As well as considering our own health and welfare as a nation, we are increasingly being involved in sharing our good fortune with third world countries. So nurses cannot be immune to the international flavour of health concern on a global basis, as our media brings far-off problems directly into our living rooms.

Two generations of Britons have been brought up entirely within the state welfare system. Whereas old people might shun the idea of 'taking charity' (which of course they are not), or will fight to retain their independence against all odds, the modern generation can get militant over their 'rights' and will make sure they get their entitlements.

Beveridge described the five freedoms to be the right of every man, woman and child: freedom from want, disease, squalor, ignorance and idleness. From these ideals was developed the welfare state, with the health service as one of the largest departments, giving everyone an opportunity for a healthy existence from the cradle to the grave, from the womb to the tomb, from hatch to despatch.

Private sector health

There is an overwhelming recognition of the benefits of the NHS, especially its egalitarian attitude, and most are keen to ensure its continued survival. Of late, the private sector of care has blossomed and attracted a lot of interest, but is largely restricted to those requiring elective surgery and, is for the most part, financed through insurance schemes. However, only the state system provides the comprehensive service that takes responsibility for critical emergencies, care of the chronically sick, aged and disabled and has the infrastructure to provide extensive community support.

Far from posing a threat to the NHS, it seems likely that the independent sector and the state service will forge links for efficient sharing of resources. This is already being done, when patients are referred, in both directions, for specialist consultation, investigation or treatment, making use of equipment available.

The move towards healthy living

People have, in the past, been fairly passive as regards their own health and treatment, not helped by professional staff who have implied that patients should remain subjugated by their better judgement and remain in a reasonable state of ignorance! In future people will be expected to take a greater responsibility for their health, both on an individual and corporate level.

There will be more emphasis on preventing disease and on personal self-reliance for remaining healthy, with less dependence on the 'nanny' state to provide all. It will be up to nurses to help people gain that interest and knowledge in health care. For, if people are well informed about health matters, they are likely to have greater respect for the service and be actively involved in its support.

There have been notable, if gradual, changes in emphasis of the health service, from its origins to current practice, as shown in Table 6.1.

Table 6.1   Changes in emphasis of the health service

From	To
Illness	Health
Treatment	Prevention
Cure	Care
Disease	Behaviour which contributes to disease
Individual treatment	Population as a unit of treatment
Hospital/institution	Community
Illness as a concern solely for professionals	Health as the business of everybody
Passive receipt/dependence	Active involvement/ independence
The right to treatment	A duty to stay healthy

Patient involvement

Healthy living is in current vogue. We are surrounded by joggers and runners, coerced into aerobic classes and beauty clubs, and encouraged to purchase whole foods from health shops.

After the postwar complacency of the 1950s and 1960s, when Britons had 'never had it so good', there came a backlash of health consciousness. This was not entirely unrelated to the awareness by the professions of the dangers of too much sugar, fat and salt, too little fibre and exercise, resulting in the western diseases of obesity, hypertension, coronary heart disease and selected cancers.

Suddenly, everyone has been bombarded to review the way they live, the food they eat and the excesses in which they indulge. Witness the exaltation of fibre, the scathing attack on processed, convenience foods, matched by the way smokers have become social pariahs.

Never a day passes without mention of some startling new theory of how to live longer or get better quality from the life you have. Fad or fact, sensational or scientific, the public can be well informed about all aspects of health, should they care to take an interest. Newspapers keep their readers up to date in trends of preventive and curative methods, while television documentaries present reasoned discussion on controversial medical and social issues.

Popular demand has swelled the market for books and magazines on diet and slimming, health and fitness, to an unprecedented number. Many books are available, explaining about medical conditions in lay terms, as well as self-help manuals for the common conditions such as depression, backache, diabetes or arthritis.

Never before have people had the *opportunity* to find out about the working of their own bodies and the administration of the health system. The information is widely available to those who choose to make use of it. No longer is health shrouded in *professional mystique*, that useful ploy devised to alienate the patient from understanding professional expertise and the use of specialist jargon that will keep the patient safely at arm's length.

Yet, not all doctors have mastered the art of talking easily to patients. It must be recognised that patients often find it difficult to assimilate complicated information at a time of emotional upheaval, when faced with a particular condition or needing surgery or investigation. It may be left to the nurse to explain what has been said in terms which the patient is able to comprehend. Considering the background of knowledge available, the patient's level of understanding may be anything on the spectrum from the well-informed and knowledgeable, through the well-intentioned, to the patient who is content to 'leave it to the doctor, he knows best'.

Nothing is more irritating for a patient than to be talked down to, when he is perfectly able to comprehend the nature of his illness. He is therefore in a good position to help himself and assist staff—this is known as patient compliance.

Informed consent

It is becoming more important to pay attention to the adequate explanation of any treatment, especially where surgery, instrumentation or anaesthesia are involved. The idea of informed consent means that the patient cannot be held legally responsible for signing his consent unless he has been made fully aware of the implications of the procedure, thoroughly explained by his doctor.

In America, where litigation has a major influence on the administration of medicine, informed consent has become big business. Doctors carry a catalogue of every imaginable complication pertaining to every operation and the percentage rates of failure and success. So, for example, the patient facing surgery on the spine will be given scientific data saying how likely the operation is to succeed in relieving the pain, the chances of backache, urinary infection and paraplegia as a side-effect. Armed with the knowledge of these risks, the patient is able to weigh up all this information and then decide if he is willing to take his chances. He thereby signs his informed consent and cannot sue if he becomes one of the unlucky statistics (provided that there is no negligence).

Although informed consent has not been taken quite so far in Britain, there have been instances where patients complained that they were not adequately informed beforehand to enable them to make a reasoned decision. The contrary argument is that people do not necessarily want to be overwhelmed with statistical data or frightened by a list of very rare possibilities.

Yet patients do want to know what is happening to them and,

certainly, professional staff are being trained to work *with* people and not simply *for* them. By implication, this means that patients are involved in their own illness and its outcome and are educated to live with their problem in the context of the community, rather than an institution.

Voluntary self-help groups

The proliferation of self-help groups, crisis groups and voluntary organisations is an encouraging sign of corporate involvement and interest in health and social problems within the community.

Groups are started either by relatives of sufferers or by veterans, those who have or are currently weathering the problem, and wish to share their unique experience with others similarly placed. Sometimes the ideas initiated and sponsored by a voluntary group assume such significance that they are adopted by the state services, such as the WRVS meals on wheels scheme, family planning clinics and the moves by NAWCH for the welfare of children in hospital.

These groups provide a central source of help, support and advice about one particular area of distress, gathering a wealth of information and understanding over many years of composite experience. They can put sufferers in touch with other members, who have been through the same ordeal, and are willing to talk about their problems and the feelings they encountered.

A self-help group can provide a much needed sense of comfort and identity, of belonging, to relieve a hollow feeling of isolation, especially after discharge from hospital, when the uncomprehending world can seem like an alien place for one who is suffering.

The examples below have been chosen to illustrate the many functions of self-help groups in general, but these by no means represent the only areas of concern of those groups mentioned, nor are they exclusive to that group.

- *Crisis support*: Samaritans; Parents Anonymous; Rape Crisis Centre; Victim Support Scheme
- *Counselling* to adapt to a changed lifestyle: Mastectomy Association; CRUSE (National Organisation for the Widowed and their Children)
- *Mutual support* for sufferer and family, especially where there is a chronic or intractable condition: Schizophrenia Fellow-

ship; Depressives Associated; Parkinson's Disease Society; Friedreich's Ataxia Group

- *Therapeutic self-help*: Anorexic Aid; Alcoholics Anonymous; Phobics Society
- *Advisory service*, to share knowledge acquired about practical methods and about aids, equipment and specialist stockists: Ileostomy Association; Mastectomy Association; Laryngectomies Club
- *Provision of facilities*, such as work centres, sheltered accommodation, holidays, education and training, trusteeship scheme, sports and recreation, respite care: PHAB (Physically Handicapped and Able Bodied); Spastics Society; ASBAH (Association for Spina Bifida and Hydrocephalus)
- *Fellowship*: Haemophilia Society; Leukaemia Society; Chemoptimists (for patients who are receiving cytotoxic drug therapy)
- *Contact* to link dispersed members: Scoliosis Self-help Group; Brittle Bone Society
- *Social interaction* with persons in a like situation: Gingerbread (one-parent families); National Association of the Childless and Childfree; Married Gay's Group
- *Information source* on specialist knowledge relating to the condition: Eczema Society; Arthritis and Rheumatism Council
- *Education of client*: National Childbirth Trust; Grapevine (sex education)
- *Education of the public and professionals*, to foster understanding and acceptance, especially where there is a need to facilitate integration into the community by influencing attitudes: Mencap (for the mentally handicapped); MIND (for the mentally ill); Spastics Society; SPOD (Sexual and Personal Relationships of the Disabled)
- *Pressure group* to improve conditions or initiate change: ASH (Action on Smoking and Health); NAWCH (National Association for the Welfare of Children in Hospital); Child Poverty Action Group
- *Fund-raising*: BLISS (Baby Life Support Systems); Imperial Cancer Research Fund
- *Research concern*: Association to Combat Huntington's Chorea; Multiple Sclerosis Society; Cystic Fibrosis Research Trust; SIDS (Sudden Infant Death Syndrome) Society

There are literally hundreds of national groups to cater for people with all manner of identifiable medical and social problems. Many have grown to an enormous size, have adopted charitable status and may hold a flag day or run charity shops to raise funds. Others may remain small because they are only serving a small population, yet it is these select few whose need is probably the greatest, as they may feel unrepresented and misunderstood elsewhere.

From the original nexus of interested people, membership swells, often to organise local functioning groups, assemble a newsletter, arrange informative meetings and gather facts about specialist shops and appliances, in order to provide helpful lists to share the expertise.

Many are keen to have interested professional health workers as associate members and find this an ideal way to get the activities of their group known to potential needy members. Most organisations are willing to contribute their considerable fund of acquired knowledge and first-hand experience to further understanding of their problem and their work amongst professional workers.

The government are also keen to foster the activities of voluntary organisations, to augment state health and social services. A nurse working in an area that has an active support group liaison would do herself and her patients a great service by finding out more about the group and making use of their facilities. For it is when patients go home that they really benefit from contact with people who have that special understanding and can truthfully say, 'I know just how you feel, it was like that for me once and this is how I coped'.

Community health council

Through their local community health council (CHC), people are encouraged to have a say about the development, management and performance of their health services. Each district has a CHC, comprising a good cross-section of representative members, some from voluntary bodies which are active locally, others from the local authority and some citizens who are simply interested in community welfare.

As the public watchdog organisation, the CHC represents the

consumer's interest in health services and guarantees that local opinion is reflected in local decisions.

It may be concerned with patient facilities, such as waiting lists, outpatient department amenities, visiting times or the standard of catering in hospitals. The CHC will express an opinion about the availability of certain services within the district, or any other amenities that may be required, or speak out if a clinic or hospital is threatened with closure.

NHS employees are excluded from membership of a CHC, so it remains an unbiased and independent body. It can hear directly from the consumer about the effectiveness of local facilities by the people who have to use them. The CHC deals with *general* complaints pertaining to standards of conditions or service, and is in no position to investigate individual complaints. It can, however, advise patients or relatives how to pursue a specific complaint through the correct channels.

Health service commissioner

The health service commissioner (HSC), also known as the Ombudsman, investigates personal complaints by aggrieved patients or relatives, who feel there has been an injustice or a failure in the service. A complaint could be levelled at a particular staff member or team, a hospital, a health authority, the ambulance service, the general practitioner or other family practitioner contractees.

The HSC does not handle any complaints that are subject to legal proceedings or dealt with by a tribunal. Neither can he question the professional decisions made by doctors and nurses with regard to individual patient care. The DHA always has prior opportunity to conduct its own local enquiry, before the HSC will embark on an investigation.

Examples of the types of cases he may handle could be concerned with lost property, accidents in hospital, poor management of a patient within an institution, poor communication, failure to impart information satisfactorily, attitudes of staff or poor provision of private patient facilities in an NHS hospital.

It is important that the NHS does have some methods of feedback as an evaluation of its performance to the consumer. Apart from the avenues described above, the new Griffiths' style management within the NHS may introduce some form of quality assessment to monitor achievement, possibly by giving questionnaires to patients for anonymous reply.

Patients do already show an interest in the running of their health service and appreciate that they have considerable influence when their voice is heard. Patients may join groups to represent the ideas of consumers at local level, or national organisations concerned with conditions and handling of patients, such as the Patients Association, AIMS (for improvement in maternity services) or the Action for Victims of Medical Accidents group.

It is also encouraging to see ex-patient participation via the League of Friends, supporting fête days and bazaars or running fund-raising exercises to boost the facilities of a local hospital.

Preventive health care

The cynics say that we run a national *illness* service, rather than a national *health* service. It is true that health care in the past has concentrated its efforts on the treatment of sickness and intervention during crisis, instead of helping people remain healthy and avoid sickness.

But the future will hopefully be geared to emphasise the preventive aspects of health care and early detection, as a cheaper and better option in the long-term. There are now many types of preventive and pre-crisis stratagems operating, aimed at detecting failing health before it presents as a full-blown illness.

The availability of computer analysis enables staff to identify vulnerable groups prone to health and social problems. This helps health workers to plan the most suitable programmes for health education, health surveillance and screening, and also to maintain regular contact with those who are at risk or in need. This may be important for isolated mothers in a deprived area, teenage pregnant girls, the elderly or handicapped or a gypsy encampment (travelling families).

From the general practitioner patient list, an age/sex register can be compiled, to alert primary care staff to groups who need follow-up, even though they may not be coming to the surgery. The health visitor can ensure that all elderly persons are screeened for eye and hearing defects, diabetes, foot problems, dietary deficiency, hypertension and anaemia, just as all children are screened through the child health clinics and school health service.

Young women are regularly seen if they attend a family planning clinic and employees may have access to an occupational health department.

The middle-aged are a group who may slip through the net of surveillance and their needs may be neglected unless they have occasion to see the doctor with a specific ailment.

Well-woman clinics

A well-woman clinic offers a wide range of screening in one visit for breast cancer, cervical cancer and gynaecological disorders, hypertension, anaemia, as well as a thorough physical examination. Similarly, there are now some *well-man clinics* offering a service to identify incipient problems before they cause damage. Private organisations offer a fee-paying service for a very comprehensive health check and preventive screening programme.

Some impressive results have been achieved by sustained and concentrated preventive measures, as shown with the improvement in dental health of the nation, antismoking campaigns, uptake of antenatal services, screening of the fetus and the neonate and, of course, the dramatic reduction in the incidence of communicable diseases via an immunisation programme.

Healthmobile

Several authorities have decided to take health care out to the people via a Healthmobile, parked centrally in a busy shopping parade or beside the local library, to offer health advice and screening. The idea of a mobile, walk-in, no wait, no booking style of clinic is immediate and effective in catching an audience, modelled on the mass X-ray units of the 1950s, which were so successful in large-scale detection of lung tuberculosis.

Many countries have chosen to link the uptake of screening and immunisation to statutory benefits: no antenatal visit, no maternity benefit; no immunisation, no child benefit. Obviously this is a way of forcing people to accept preventive health care but it is a passive acceptance on an automatic level.

It is perhaps preferable to educate the public to understand the sense behind the services available, so they can make a positive decision and judge for themselves how best to take care of their bodies.

Health education

Health education is the key to preventive care in the United Kingdom, while uptake of recommendations and facilities is central to its success. Otherwise you are left with 'you can take a horse to water but you can't make it drink'.

Any positive health programme needs active participation from the clients, who must be encouraged to be self-reliant and take a pride in good health. Education should supply them with an interest and understanding, to feel that they are doing themselves some good, that their visit is worthwhile and necessary.

People must be encouraged and given the opportunity to seek help when they anticipate problems, rather than waiting for a crisis. At present, patients do feel they need to muster some reasonable symptoms of ill-health in order to qualify for a visit to the doctor. There is much more need for a counselling and advisory role, as demonstrated by the health visitor and GP practice nurse.

People must also recognise that every mental, physical and emotional ill cannot be assuaged by popping a pill into the mouth, that some pain, anxiety, grief, depression and disappointment are all part of life's rich pattern.

The preventive and educative role has traditionally been the domain of health visitors, the school nurse and the occupational health nurse, whose work centres on this aspect of care. However, they no longer have this sole prerogative, because health education becomes the responsibility of every health worker and is certainly a large component of all nurse training programmes. Wherever her occupation takes her, the nurse can develop her potential as regards education about healthy living.

Interested lay groups might ask health care professionals to talk about different aspects of their work, and nurses should welcome the opportunity to share useful information to a captive audience, whether it be a group of pregnant women at antenatal class, a church group or an invitation to a National Housewives Register group.

Health education commences with the very young and there is a lot of input with schoolchildren on dental hygiene, hand washing and handling of food, sex education and family planning.

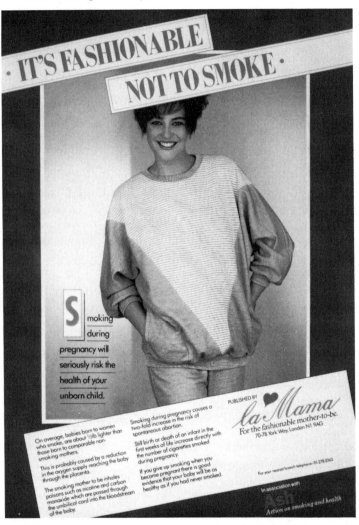

Fig. 6.2   An example of a company, la Mama, and a campaigning group, ASH, working together for health education. (Reproduced by kind permission of la Mama Ltd.)

Health education unit

Most DHAs have a central information and resource area, in the form of a health education unit, run by a district education officer. She can issue films, leaflets and provide up-to-date information for use by employees within the district, with the particular emphasis on health education and preventive methods.

Commercial companies give financial backing to the production of instructional material, loosely based to promote their product but with a true informative component.

Health Education Council (HEC)

The Health Education Council (HEC) is a national body, financially supported by DHSS and other funding, with a variety of responsibilities related to advice and instruction on general matters of health for the public. The Council has been responsible for many campaigns to promote aspects of healthy living, such as reducing smoking generally in the population, and particularly in pregnant women, alerting the public to the dangers of alcohol and drug abuse, as well as recommendations for a balanced diet and regular exercise, in order to achieve the optimum level of health. The aim is towards the correction of faulty habits within the individual, the family and the general society, as well as bringing to public notice available services.

Advertising through media channels, such as TV, radio and magazines or newspapers, is used to good effect to stimulate interest in health care ideas and facilities.

The patient's day

If a patient is admitted using a nursing care plan, he will have the opportunity to talk about his problem, to tell the nurse of his likes, dislikes, preferences and special needs. He can establish a rapport with the nurse in charge of his care and feel free to discuss any anxieties in relation to his admission.

As a rule, patients are no longer woken at the crack of dawn for the daily temperature round, which can easily be done in the afternoon, but are allowed to take a leisurely breakfast when the day staff come on duty.

The majority of hospitals are able to offer their patients a choice of menu for each meal, with a selection from two hot meals and a salad as alternative, and a hot sweet or fruit. Large, medium or small portions can be requested.

Each patient fills a daily menu sheet for the following day, assisted by the ward clerk or receptionist. Meals are dished out in the kitchen and the completed trays are delivered to the ward as a plated meals service, which requires no serving by ward staff.

Hospital design has tended to move away from the long Nightingale ward and wards are now split into bays containing four, six or eight beds, sometimes with a mixed sex allocation of patients. This facilitates better use of bed complement, as bays can be allocated to either men or women, depending on the current need.

Newer hospitals often have the racetrack design, with ward bays down either side of the circular corridor, and the nurses' station, examination room and utilities placed centrally.

Each bedspace is fitted with a call system, which registers at the central station, and newly built hospitals are equipped with piped oxygen and suction apparatus to each space.

As patients are encouraged to be up and out of bed more quickly these days, many are encouraged to wear day clothes when they feel better, rather than stay in pyjamas or dressing gown. A day room is a useful feature for patients who like to escape from their bed in the ward, and sit in comfort watching the television, having their meals sitting at a communal table and entertaining visitors.

Most hospitals have dispensed with the traditional formal visiting hour and have moved towards more flexible visiting times. This is not the same as open or unrestricted visiting, as found on children's wards, where parents are allowed to come at any time of the day or night. Flexible visiting permits visitors at times which suit the schedule of the patient and the ward, generally excluding meal times, clinical procedures, examinations and treatments, doctor's rounds and designated rest periods.

Visiting is usually between 2 pm and 8 pm, and allows visitors to come at any time during that period, to suit their other commitments. They may stay for as long—or as short—a duration as they like, at the discretion of the nurse in charge, who will know how much the patient can comfortably tolerate. It obviates that dreadful prolonged hour, when visitors run out of conversation or the patient is feeling tired and strained, yet both feel obliged to sit it out until the bell sanctions their departure.

As an added measure of safety, each patient who is admitted to hospital, including day cases and newly born babies delivered on the premises, has a personalised identiband attached to his wrist. This is a strip of card, bearing details of full name, age, ward, hospital number, encased in a plastic cover. This is securely clipped to the wrist, is impervious to water and can only be removed by cutting the plastic. Details must be checked by two nurses, as this forms the definitive identification of the patient, used when giving drugs, a blood transfusion or prior to surgery, when using a preoperative checklist.

Various alternative terms are used to describe people on the receiving end of care. 'Patient' is the one used in hospital, and for people who are having medical or nursing attention because they are ill. 'Client' is used by social service personnel and by people such as health visitors working with the non-ill. 'Resident' is the preferred term when people are living in some kind of institution, hostel or community home. Increasingly the term 'consumer' is being adopted and, although it has financial connotations, it recognises the position of the person as being in receipt of a service. And more and more there is the view that the service should be geared to the patient's specific needs, rather than expecting him to grab what he can from a rigid schedule.

With the proper use of individualised patient care, it would be hoped that ward activity accommodates to what the patient wants, rather than adheres to a blind routine. For example, the rheumatoid patient might like an early warm bath to ease his stiffened joints, whereas the surgical patient may prefer to take his time and bath later in the day. Nurses themselves need to adapt to the style of individualised patient care, which is central to current nursing practice.

Reference and refresher reading

Gaffin J. (ed.) (1981). *The Nurse and the Welfare State.* Aylesbury: HM and M Publishers.
National Council of Voluntary Organisations (1984–85). *The National Council of Voluntary Organisations Directory.* London: Bedford Square

Press: A most useful handbook listing all the current voluntary organisations.

Strehlow M. S. (1984). *Education for Health: A Guide for Health Visitors, Nurses and All Others Working in the Community*. London: Harper and Row.

7

Current Nursing Practice

The modern philosophy of the nursing process is based upon individualised patient care, making use of systematised planning to deliver specific care to suit the needs of each patient.

The nursing model of care

Before attempting to implement any nursing strategy for patient care, it is necessary to recognise what is required for that person from a nursing standpoint, and how these needs are best likely to be met.

The medical model of care seeks information about signs, symptoms and the results of investigations about an illness, attempts to make a diagnosis, and then institutes treatment for that condition. This approach is disease-oriented.

A nursing model obviously takes cognisance of the medical condition but focuses its attention on the all-round functioning of the individual. The role of the nurse is to help the patient to re-cover and regain the maximum level of independence.

For example, the doctor will diagnose bronchitis and prescribe antibiotics and physiotherapy, whereas the nurse will assess how the bronchitis affects his ability to breathe, to eat, to sleep, to move, etc. This approach is problem-oriented, concentrating on the difficulties the patient experiences as a result of the illness, and examines how these can be alleviated by nursing action.

There are several theoretical models of nursing care and the one shown in Table 7.1 has been devised by Roper, Logan and

Table 7.1   The activities of living model of nursing

Maintaining a safe environment	Controlling body temperature
Communicating	Mobilising
Breathing	Working and playing
Eating and drinking	Expressing sexuality
Eliminating waste matter	Sleeping
Personal cleansing and dressing	Dying

Tierney (1980). It is based upon the twelve activities of living (AL), which must be considered when trying to identify the needs of patients and to plan a programme of nursing care.

When using the holistic approach to nursing care, the nurse takes account of all the factors in a person's makeup that make him a unique individual. She considers the physical, emotional, intellectual, social and spiritual aspects affecting the disease process, relating both to its causation and to its outcome.

The nursing process

The nursing process is the theoretical framework for the development of patient care planning. Using the nursing care plan as the basic tool to devise a programme, a personalised plan of care is tailored for each individual patient. The principle is founded on a problem-solving approach, working in four progressive steps: assessment, planning, implementation and evaluation (see Figure 7.1).

Use of the nursing process encourages nurses to think for themselves, use their initiative, make reasoned decisions and undertake responsibility for patient care. It also leads to greater appreciation of the patient as a unique individual and an understanding of the variables within human existence.

Learners benefit by being involved early on in the total care of patients. Patients also appear to respond favourably to a greater rapport with one or two members of the nursing staff, who have developed a close interest in their special needs.

Assessment

Each patient has a *nursing history* taken on admission, in order to assess his general condition and normal lifestyle. In addition to information gathered from the patient and relative during an informal interview, the nurse's own observations are important, such as whether he looks obese, dehydrated, anxious or depressed.

The nursing history data sheets, shown in Figures 7.2 and 7.3, are self-explanatory. They request information that will help complete a picture of the patient in order that the nurse can plan a care programme appropriate for his unique needs. Dietary likes and dislikes, the degree of mobility, allergies, aids for seeing,

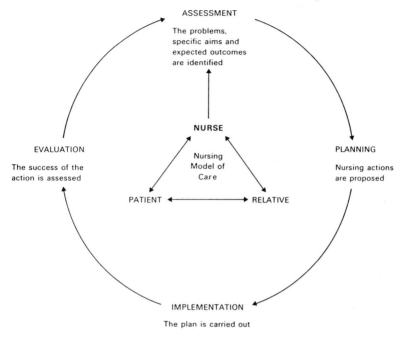

Fig. 7.1 The cycle of the nursing process.

hearing and moving, religion, language, family circumstances and employment, together with the physical and emotional state, are necessary facts to build up a visual image of that individual.

The information should be collected and recorded sometime during the day of admission by the admitting nurse, who is also responsible for his orientation to the ward and neighbouring patients, plus routine observations.

One section which asks, 'patient's reason for admission', is important for establishing why he thinks he is in hospital and how much he knows about his condition. 'Waterworks trouble', for instance, could mean kidney disease, cystitis or an enlarged prostate.

Taking a history should be done privately, in confidence, as an unhurried procedure, where the patient is encouraged to talk and the nurse to listen carefully. This permits a two-way communication between the nurse and patient, nurse and relative, allowing each to ask questions about hospitalisation and forthcoming management.

Nursing History

NAME Mrs. Ellen LYME,
ADDRESS 15 Winchester Lane,
Ottersbury,
LYMSHIRE J.

D.O.B. 1-6-20

(AFFIX ADDRESSOGRAPH LABEL)

PATIENTS TELEPHONE No. 023-65609

DATE & TIME OF ADMISSION 3.9.85 14.00 hrs.

RE-ADMISSION DATE & TIME

BOOKED/A & E/TRANSFER/OPD Daughter

RELATIVES INFORMED YES NO accompanied Daughter

MARITAL STATUS Widow

RELIGION C/E

G.P Dr. Pond,

ADDRESS 43 Field Street,
Ottersbury,
LYMSHIRE.

NEXT OF KIN (NAME) Mrs. Pat Cox

RELATIONSHIP TO PATIENT Daughter

ADDRESS 15 Winchester Lane
Ottersbury,
LYMSHIRE.

TEL. No HOME 023-65609
WORK 023-214-28 (ext 212)

OTHER RELATIVE (NAME) Mr. Alan Cox

RELATIONSHIP TO PATIENT Son-in-law

ADDRESS 15 Winchester Lane.
Ottersbury,
LYMSHIRE.

TEL. No HOME 023-65609
WORK 023-5629 1 (ext 33)

PATIENT'S REASON FOR ADMISSION

Fears it is a stroke

PATIENT AWARE OF DIAGNOSIS YES NO

RELATIVES AWARE OF DIAGNOSIS YES NO

RELATIVES SEEN BY MEDICAL STAFF YES NO   DATES SEEN   3.9.85.

INFORMATION GIVEN TO PATIENT

3.9.85. Told she has probably had a stroke and would need to remain in hospital for a while

10.9.85. Progressing well enough to be prepared for discharge.

DIAGNOSIS Right-sided cerebro-vascular accident.
Left hemiplegia

HISTORY OF PRESENT COMPLAINT

Woke from a doze, unable to move left hand or leg, and difficulty in swallowing.
Speech intact.

OTHER CURRENT HEALTH PROBLEMS AND MEDICATIONS

Osteo-arthritis in back and left hip.
Indocid t.d.s.

ALLERGIES   PENICILLIN

PAST MEDICAL HISTORY/OPERATIONS

Right hip replacement 1982

SOCIAL

OCCUPATION School Dinner Lady PRESENT/RETIRED

CHILDREN One daughter AGES (IF UNDER 16)

OTHER DEPENDANTS

ACCOMMODATION Lives with daughter and son-in-laws

CARE AT HOME   DETAILS

COMMUNITY NURSE

HEALTH VISITOR

SOCIAL WORKER

SOCIAL SERVICES
(Please specify)   N/A   3.9.85.

CONSULTANT   DR. SMETHWICK

NAME   MRS. Ellen LYME

Fig 7.2 A nursing history sheet (from St Vincent's Orthopaedic Hospital, Pinner, Middlesex)

DIET

SPECIAL

FOOD DISLIKES Liver and Kidney

DRINK DISLIKES Coffee

SMOKER [NON SMOKER]

APPETITE [GOOD] POOR

ORAL
OWN TEETH Upper
DENTURES UPPER /[LOWER]
CROWNS
REMARKS Own teeth in poor condition

HEARING
GOOD /[POOR]/ DEAF
HEARING AID YES /[NO]
REMARKS Embarrassed at being hard of hearing.
ANY SPEECH DIFFICULTY Slurred speech since C.V.A.
LANGUAGE SPOKEN English

VISION
[GOOD]
PARTIALLY SIGHTED
REGISTERED BLIND
REMARKS Wears glasses for reading

MOBILITY
HOW MOBILE Limited through arthritis.
ANY PARALYSIS Left hemiplegia
ANY PROSTHESIS Right hip prosthesis
AIDS REQUIRED Uses a walking stick.
HELP REQUIRED
LEFT /[RIGHT HANDED]

REMARKS Normally has a limp, but confined to bed rest at present.

MENSTRUAL HISTORY (IF RELEVANT)
DATE OF L.M.P. N/A
PILL YES/NO

REMARKS

BOWELS
(ANY PROBLEMS) Regular daily action.

MEDICATION (IF ANY) —

BLADDER
(ANY PROBLEMS) Needs to pass urine once during the night.
CATHETER IN SITU YES /[NO]
DATE LAST CHANGED

NAME Mrs. Ellen LYME

SLEEP

HOW MANY HOURS USUALLY 6
SEDATION NONE

REMARKS Usually wakes early

NURSES OBSERVATIONS Independent lady

MENTAL ATTITUDE Brave and optimistic outlook. Anxious not to become a "burden".

GENERAL APPEARANCE Looks in good health
[NORMAL]/ OBESE / THIN / EMACIATED / DEHYDRATED / ACUTELY ILL

SKIN Slightly dry

BROKEN AREAS (DESCRIBE) None

OTHER REMARKS Toenails in need of attention. ? See visiting chiropodist

LEVEL OF CONSCIOUSNESS (REMARKS) Conscious and orientated to her surroundings.

T 36.4 P 96 R 18 B/P 170/100 WT 67kg HT 1.60

URINALYSIS N.A.D.

VALUABLES AND HOW STORED Yellow metal ring (Left hand) and watch retained by patient.

ANY OTHER USEFUL INFORMATION
Is on orthopaedic waiting list for right hip replacement repeat and to failed prosthesis.

INFORMATION OBTAINED FROM Mrs Lyme + Mrs. Cox
BY St. J/N. T. Wentworth
DATE 3.9.85.

CONSULTANT DR. SMETHWICK

NR 2

Fig. 7.3 The daily living sheet.

DATE	INVESTIGATIONS/OPERATIONS	DATE	REMINDERS
3.9.85.	E.C.G. ✓ CXR Portable ✓	8.9.85	Try big bath today ✓
5.9.85.	M.S.U. ✓	9.9.85	Speak to relatives re discharge ✓
7.9.86.	Repeat CXR ✓	10.9.85.	See visiting chiropodist ✓
		11.9.85	Ask relatives to bring clothes

DISCHARGE PLANNING

PLANNED DATE OF DISCHARGE 14.9.85.

	Needed	Date Ordered	Date to Commence
SOCIAL SERVICES (SPECIFY)	✓	12.9.85.	13.9.85.
COMMUNITY NURSE	✓	12.9.85	
TTA'S AND INSTRUCTION			
TRANSPORT	relative's transport		
RELATIVES INFORMED	✓	12.9.85	
OUT-PATIENT APPOINTMENT	✓	12.9.85	27.10.85
LETTER TO G.P.	✓	12.9.85	Sent
VALUABLES RETURNED	retained by patient during admission		

SIGNATURE J. Heartwell

DATE	PATIENT'S PROBLEMS/NEEDS	AIMS	ACTION	EVALUATION/DATE
3.9.85.	A) Hypertension	Reduce high blood pressure.	Bedrest 4 hourly B.P. Medication as prescribed.	5.9.85. B.P. reduced and controlled. May mobilise gradually
	B) Bedrest for 24 hours	Prevent complications of Deep Vein Thrombosis, Chest Infection, Pressure Sores.	Alternate position 2 hourly. Leg and deep breathing exercises. Pressure area care.	5.9.85. Sitting out in chair. N.B. sore areas on skin
	C) Personal hygiene	Maintain cleanliness and comfort.	Daily bed bath. Help with oral hygiene, hair care and using bedpans.	7.9.85 Help with washing at sink. P.Bhm
	D) Difficulty with eating and drinking	Maintain fluid and nutritional requirements. Prevent urinary infection.	2 hourly fluid of 200 mls. Use of non-slip mat, scoop bowl.	5.9.85. Intake tolerated well

		Soft diet and help with feeding.	
E) Paralysis of left side.	Regain maximum functional ability.	Daily physiotherapy. Passive and active exercises.	6.9.85. Regaining use of left limbs. 7-9-85. Using tripod. P.S.
F) Slurring of speech.	Restore speech.	Reassurance and give opportunity to practise talking.	7-9-85. Speech much improved. P.Smm
G) Painful arthritic joints.	Relieve pain.	N.S.A.I. drugs as prescribed.	5.9.85. Pain well controlled.

NAME Mrs. Ellen LYME ⁷/⁹⁵ CONSULTANT DR. SMETHWICK NR 2

Fig. 7.4 The planned programme of care.

Using the data gathered from the nursing history, enables the nurse to identify special problems affecting this patient, sometimes called a *nursing diagnosis*.

Problems which require urgent attention may already be present, such as shortness of breath or pain. Or problems can be foreseen as potential hazards, such as pressure sores for someone confined to bed, or infection in an open wound.

It is important to find out what the patient can and cannot do for himself, or establish any mechanisms he uses to help him manage his difficulties, such as choosing to sleep upright on pillows or having analgesia prior to exercise.

Planning

Having identified a problem, the nurse should be able to specify her ultimate aim: either to alleviate an actual problem or prevent a potential one. The planned action of nursing intervention is intended to fulfil these aims. Goals must be realistic and adjusted to take account of the abilities and resources of that patient. For example, the goal for mobility will be vastly different for a young man having an appendicectomy, compared to an octogenarian amputee having suffered a stroke. Figure 7.4 shows a planned programme of nursing care.

The planning should, whenever possible, be done in conjunction with the patient, to ensure his understanding and compliance with the programme. Final decisions are corroborated by the nurse in charge, especially when learners are involved in care planning. For example: *potential problem* is risk of pressure sores; *aim* is to keep skin dry and clean, to prevent redness and soreness; *plan of action* would be two-hourly turning, provision of sheepskin pad and bootees.

This method is repeated to take account of all problems through every aspect of daily living and may be listed as numbers or alphabetical letters for easy reference without unnecessary repetition of writing.

Implementation

After preparing the care plan, the nurse will carry out the actions of nursing intervention proposed regarding the management of the patient. When specific care has been prescribed, such as two-hourly turning, it is important that the nurse signs when it is completed, with the date and time of each entry.

Evaluation

Evaluation is a necessary part of the continuing plan of care, vital in judging how effective the action has been. Has the aim been achieved, and the action appropriate? If it has not been successful, the action may need to be reassessed, with a change or modification subsequently.

If the patient at risk from pressure sores will not remain turned on one side and there is evidence of redness of the skin, use of a ripple mattress may be required.

For the postoperative patient, hourly observations may be reduced to two-hourly, then four-hourly, once the patient's condition has stabilised.

Kardex system

The Kardex (card index) system comprises forms upon which all current and relevant patient information is recorded and stored. It replaces all previous miscellaneous books which used to record patient care tasks, such as bathing, urine testing, dressings, temperature and bowel action.

A Kardex is both a permanent record and legal document, so that entries should be written legibly, with the minimum of accepted abbreviations and signed by each nurse who attends the patient. It must be accessible to all nurses at all times, preferably kept at the nurses' station, as it is the definitive reference and only written source of the patient and his particular needs.

One sheet records data of nursing history and another activities of living. A separate sheet records the four sections of the nursing care plan and includes space to record special instruction, such as dates of operations, investigations and examinations, and reminders. As Figure 7.4 shows, another space is for discharge planning, which should be organised in advance to prepare outside agencies for forthcoming responsibilities.

Patients continue to have separate charts for observations, fluid intake and output and a drug record.

There is no national Kardex form, and each authority will adopt one specifically to suit its own use. Indeed, they may devise several forms to cater for diverse situations where needs vary, such as day surgery, paediatrics, psychiatry or community care.

Patient-centred allocation

Of fundamental importance to the success of the nursing process is that one nurse is responsible for the total patient care during one span of duty. This is known as patient-centred allocation or patient assignment.

The senior ward nurse, as team leader, will allocate a number of patients to a nurse, taking account of the ward workload, levels of dependency of patients and experience of the nurse. In a high-dependency situation like intensive care units, this may be a 1:1 nurse:patient ratio, but on a general ward the nurse would care for several patients.

Using the programmes of planned care, the nurse will attend to the needs of each of her charges, complete the nursing records and charts and hand over the report to her colleague on the next shift. Although she may be unable to do everything for each patient, if for example one of her patients had to be accompanied to another department for an investigation, she takes overall responsibility that the care has been completed. Obviously nurses will need to cooperate with each other when needing help with patient care or taking a mealbreak.

Ideally the nurse should maintain continuity of care, by looking after the same patients when she returns to duty, giving her the opportunity to follow patient care through from admission to discharge.

The nurse in charge of the ward acts as leader and coordinator, to give guidance and advice, as she delegates many of her traditional duties to the nurse responsible for the patient's total care. For example, only a nurse knowing the patient, his condition and management, should accompany the doctors' round, to report on behalf of that patient. She will also be responsible for arranging any appointments or investigations pertinent for her patients.

Patient allocation is a method designed to give the patients' needs top priority, rather than a sterile list of tasks executed in a rigid ward routine, timed solely to suit the organisation.

This method contrasts with the old *task-centred allocation* or job assignment, where nurses were given a series of chores to complete on a ward-round basis. Tasks were meted out according to a level of ability in the hierarchy, with juniors circulating to take temperatures and give bedpans, while seniors prepared surgical patients, gave out drugs and did dressings, and trained staff had the accolade of joining the doctors' rounds.

This system resulted in fragmentary care that did not often fit in with the patient's needs, with little continuity of personalised attention, leaving the patient to call upon any available member of staff passing by who happened to be free. With patient-centred allocation, the patient knows who is looking after him at any one time and to whom he should refer, thus improving the line of communication.

Nurses used to be assigned to boring repetitious routines, with the final responsibility of pulling the strings together to collate all aspects of care resting with the sister in charge. Patient allocation means that junior nurses are introduced to the full spectrum of integrated nursing care at an early stage, working alongside a senior nurse to whom she can refer. They learn to be inquiring, question their decisions and take responsibility, as they plan and execute a programme of care. And this they find more satisfying and of greater benefit as preparation for being a qualified nurse.

Patient-centred allocation also keeps senior nurses at the bedside, involved in the job for which they were trained, rather than delegating 'basic' tasks to junior staff.

With the emphasis on technological achievements assisting patient care, a nurse may find herself paying more attention to 'nursing the machines' and undermining the essential basic needs of the patient. She may even lose sight of the person underneath, who is alienated as something of a physiological entity without feelings and personality.

It is a welcome reappraisal of values in the profession that down-to-earth 'hands-on care', of vital importance to the patient, is making a comeback. A topical phrase describing the whole concept of individualised patient care is 'rediscovering the patient'.

Criticism of the nursing process

The acceptance and implementation of the nursing process has not altogether had a smooth passage into the profession, and has not been without its critics. It was ushered in by enthusiastic academics as a theoretical model, which had difficulty becoming established as a meaningful practical tool with relevance to working nurses and sick patients.

Much of the initial problem was in feeling constrained by preset printed plans of care, which did not equate with the needs for all nursing occasions. The nursing process, in fact, should be flexible, open to adaptation and evolution through use and practice.

Some authorities employed a senior nurse specifically to introduce the nursing process and its practical application to employees in the district. Called a 'patient care planning coordinator' or a similar term, it was her task to get the idea adopted at the grass roots level. She would explain the philosophy to groups of staff and devise plans for different fields of care, while always adhering to the principles of the nursing process.

The use of the nursing process may fail due to three basic causes.

(1) If the nursing history and care plan are just seen as another set of forms, to be duly completed and filed away, without taking due heed of the information given. One example is of the mother admitted with her child, who was very impressed at the questions on the history and duly reported that her son was allergic to eggs. She was therefore understandably disappointed that a boiled egg was served without fail every morning! This makes a nonsense of asking for the facts in the first place.

(2) Without patient allocation, nurses continue circulating on task rounds of care and have no specific responsibility or rapport with particular patients. However, it must be said that this is difficult to implement when there is a shortage of staff, particularly trained staff to supervise the care plans. With one staff nurse and one auxiliary covering a ward of 25 patients on the evening shift, care is relegated to priority needs and expeditious completion of routine tasks only.

(3) The nursing process stands no chance at all if it is greeted with open hostility and a wall of rejection, and dismissed as a new-fangled device sent to upset the cosy routines of nurses set in their ways.

Returning nurses could be excused for thinking that the nursing process is old-style care wrapped up in new-style jargon, with a lot of added paperwork. No one can deny that the fundamentals of care are the same, but the systematised personal approach should lead to improved communication and integration of activities.

As the nursing process is increasingly used with effect, it is proving beneficial for both patient care and job satisfaction for nurses.

The nurse's role in patient education

A nurse has the unique distinction of being directly and fully involved in patient care around the clock. She is accessible and is therefore ideally placed to educate the patient about his condition and management of related aspects, either formally or informally.

Patient education is such a fundamental role for the nurse, that teaching skills are incorporated in nurse training programmes. Indeed, the concept of the nursing process expects the patient to be involved through understanding in his own planned programme of care, to ensure his cooperation and compliance.

Within the patient population, knowledge and comprehension of medical matters varies enormously and the nurse must learn to pitch her style, depth and language at an appropriate level. She must also be aware of the emotions which interfere with acceptance of information, that hospitalisation itself is a fearful and alien environment for many and a source of great anxiety.

Patient education can be anything from a casual enquiry at the bedside to a formal teaching session with a group.

Provider of information

The one resounding complaint from patients is the lack of information given in hospital, especially surrounding forthcoming tests and surgery. It is as if the staff are so used to doing routine procedures that they forget that it may be the first time for the patient, who has no idea what to expect. As the person caring for the patient, the nurse should ensure that he is sufficiently informed throughout his stay and given the opportunity to ask questions.

On admission, a notable time for a high level of anxiety, he should be given information pertaining to the hospital and ward—visiting times, meals, hospital shop, telephoning arrangements—and generally made to feel that his inquiries are welcomed.

Although it is the doctor's responsibility to explain about the patient's condition and surgical details in order to get the consent signed, the nurse acts as a backup in this respect. It never hurts to go over what has been said in an informal way, allowing the patient to absorb the information and get it clear in his mind. The patient may not have understood what the doctor said but was embarrassed to trouble him further, or perhaps he thought of a question later. The nurse may well find herself in the role of 'translator'.

She must also try to anticipate what the patient should need to know in preparation for future events. To say 'you are having an operation on your stomach', says little to the patient who has never had surgery before. It is up to the nurse to acquaint him with what to expect: the anaesthetic, feeling drowsy and dry in the mouth; the nasogastric tube; the infusion of blood into one arm; nausea and pain, which can be relieved. Patients are often alarmed to wake up and find all kinds of paraphernalia on and emitting from them, which signals disaster in their minds but is in fact all routine: 'forewarned is forearmed'.

Some startling research findings have shown how beneficial and effective preoperative preparation can be. Those patients who were given good, sensible information before their operation showed less anxiety, needed less postoperative analgesia and made quicker progress to recovery with less complications.

If patients are to be transferred to the intensive care unit after surgery or placed in isolation, it is helpful if the staff can visit the patient beforehand, so that he will recognise a friendly face and establish a link with his carer.

In the future we may see video-recordings describing operation details and postoperative management, in order to allow patients to be prepared before they undergo booked surgery.

Teacher and adviser

Teaching involves helping someone to acquire the knowledge and skills he will need, in order to understand about his condition and how best to manage it. Every health visitor does this kind of teaching with expectant mothers in an antenatal class, to prepare for the birth of their children.

For example, the patient with diabetes will need to understand how diet and insulin work, how important it is to adhere to the carefully planned regime, and to know the signs when things go wrong.

Colitis, diverticulitis, arthritis, eczema and asthma are examples of chronic conditions that are suffered without hospitalisation, so the patient needs advice and encouragement to cope in day-to-day existence.

Many hospitals now issue advice sheets for patients to take home, to continue their progress after discharge, such as a back pain programme or postnatal exercises or care of a plaster of Paris (see Figure 7.5).

Also important is advice on discharge following any kind of surgery, with a list of the type of questions the patient may think of later at home. People who are concentrating on survival and getting back on their feet rarely think beyond the hospital gates. It is not until they are discharged that they realise they had forgotten to ask questions like: When can I drive? When can I resume sexual relations? Should I go walking or swimming or play golf? Can I take alcohol? These affect all patients whether having a gynaecological operation, hip replacement or heart surgery.

Instructor

There are many instances where a nurse must be involved in demonstrating manipulative or social skills and supervising practice, to help a patient master a technique. The midwife does this when she gives parentcraft classes to new mothers, as does the nurse in mental handicap work, training her clients to shop and cook, or to handle fares on public transport. For example, a new diabetic patient would need to learn precisely how to prepare a syringe of insulin and to inject it into the appropriate site.

Patients being discharged on medication must be given very clear instructions about the dose and time of the drug and the side-effects to watch for. This is particularly important for those on steroid or anticoagulant therapy. Where multiple drugs are prescribed, especially for the elderly who get confused, a record of administration chart should be given, which also doubles as a checklist to see if the drugs have been taken.

When patients are discharged in plaster of Paris, they must be

---

Instructions Given to all Out-Patients Leaving with Plasters

Out-patients must be given written *as well as verbal instructions* and the nurse must make sure that these are understood. Most A & E departments ask their patients to return the following day for a 'plaster check'.

1. Instruct the patient to compare digits of the unplastered limb to check that all is well on the plastered one. Should the plastered fingers or toes become *blue, white, cold,* or *swollen* or become *painful, numb* or feel like '*pins and needles*', report to your doctor or the hospital without delay.

2. During the first few days after application, do not let the plaster hang down unless in active use. Keep the limb *elevated* on a *soft* surface, cushions, pillows, armsling.

3. Practise the exercises you have been shown at least three times daily and exercise joints which have not been immobilised in plaster. Once the plaster is dry, general use is recommended.

4. If you feel a 'blister-like' *burning pain* under the plaster or if there is any *unpleasant odour* or *discharge* from inside the cast, contact your doctor or hospital.

5. If a child *drops any object*, such as a coin or pencil under the plaster this could be responsible for producing a sore and should be reported immediately.

6. If the plaster becomes *loose, cracked* or *soft*, report back to the hospital to have it inspected.

7. *Avoid* getting the plaster *wet*.

Fig. 7.5   *An example of patient education.*

given precise instructions by the nurse, both verbal and written, about the care of the plaster, observation of the digits, and return appointment.

Counsellor

In counselling, the nurse helps the patient to explore all avenues of the problem, in order that *he* can make *his* decision from among the many choices available. She does not aim to direct or influence the patient's decision, although she may be able to clarify the alternatives.

She does not sit in moral judgement, nor suggest what she herself would choose to do, for she has a different set of circumstances, personality and opinions.

The nurse cannot answer for someone else who is faced with cancer of the bowel versus a colostomy, nor for a pregnant woman who has found out that her fetus has a defect.

In an understanding atmosphere, the patient is allowed to draw on his own resources and acts as he thinks appropriate in the light of his situation.

Social workers often like to think they have the sole prerogative in the role of counselling but, in reality, patients will seek out the person to whom they wish to talk, this being the nurse who is available. But if she does enter into the counselling role, the nurse must be very careful not to be drawn to make a decision for the patient who is in a quandary.

Counselling may also be concerned with adjustment to a new situation, such as bereavement, living with paralysis, or the loss of a breast or other part of the body.

Advocate

The complete opposite of counsellor is the role of advocate—this means that one person speaks on behalf of another who is unable to represent himself or his own interests.

This could be most obviously applied in caring for the mentally ill or mentally handicapped, who may need a professional person to represent their best interests and speak on their behalf.

Yet in any field of nursing the patient is always the focal point of the nurse's work and it is to his ultimate benefit that all her energies must be committed. In practice, nurses frequently speak for their patient's wellbeing when he is unable to do so, by getting the best management for him, by helping and supporting him and bringing him into contact with suitable agencies and personnel. Advocacy is inherent in the nurse's role.

Extended role

Much is now talked of the extended role of the qualified nurse, as her work increasingly brings her into contact with high-powered technical skills, formerly the exclusive responsibility of doctors.

Although everyone would resist the notion of nurses adopting the mini-doctor role, there are some clinical situations where it is sensible to extend the responsibility of the nurse and add to her skills. In any crisis it is the nurse who is first at hand on the scene and she could use her advanced skills for effective and immediate action.

In the intensive care unit, where time is critical and waiting to bleep a doctor could be the difference between life and death, nurses are taught to interpret ECG readings, take venous blood, use a defibrillator and to add drugs to established intravenous lines. Likewise, nurses working in accident and emergency departments are taught to suture wounds and to pass an endotracheal tube, as are those working in the anaesthetic room or with premature babies in special care baby units.

It would be professionally irresponsible and illegal for a nurse to attempt *any* procedure for which she has not been *adequately trained* and is *legally not entitled* to perform.

Techniques which are part of the extended role are not included in the basic training programmes and are not, as such, acknowledged by the registering body of the UKCC. Many, as described above, are incorporated into the specialist post-basic clinical nursing courses and training is given by the training establishment.

At present, the employing authority defines the qualifying mechanism which enables trained nurses to perform these duties within their district. This usually comprises training in theory and method, supervised practice, and a certificate legally covering the nurse to undertake this technique and covering the authority who is allowing her to do so. A nurse would not have a leg to stand on if she acted without the proper credentials and something went seriously wrong.

Even though a nurse has been certified competent by one authority, she may need to get another local authorisation should she be working in a different district, to continue to be legally covered in performing these duties.

Accountability and the law

As professional people, nurses are liable in law for their independent actions. When assuming a greater role in the decision-making process, she must be accountable for the responsibility of her performance in a professional capacity. Just as doctors can be asked to validate a certain choice of treatment, so the nurse can expect to account for her plan of nursing care.

Nurses have a responsibility to deliver to patients care of the highest possible standard, which is safe, moral, caring and effective. It is therefore necessary to adhere to both parts of the nursing process: to state the expected outcome of nursing intervention, and to evaluate the result. In this respect, she can account for her actions and discard any practices which prove ineffective.

To be accountable for one's actions presupposes an adequate level of knowledge and competence to take on this responsibility. This is where training and assessment of the learner are necessary before awarding a qualification which admits a nurse to the profession. In the United Kingdom, every nurse is bound by law, which gives the public protection from illegal and inept practitioners, as laid down in the Nurses, Midwives and Health Visitors Act of 1979. The UKCC and the four national boards are empowered by statute to uphold the standards of conduct of the profession, to monitor the training and registration of all practitioners in nursing, midwifery and health visiting.

It is imperative that nurses be conversant with the law, as it relates to them as employees, as practitioners and as members of the general society. Some laws are directly related to a nurse's practice, such as administration of drugs, patients' consent to treatment, midwives delivering babies and action under the laws pertaining to mental health.

Some are not so clearly defined, such as notification of accidents, self-discharge, handling a rape victim, and the complaints procedure. Instructions for local interpretation and administration are to be found in the District Policies and Procedures File, one of which should be available in each ward and department. Every nurse should acquaint herself with local policies at her place of work, as part of her contract of employment.

The need to maintain clear, accurate and updated nursing records cannot be emphasised too strongly, as these constitute legal documents and can be summoned for examination during any formal enquiry.

Management

Management has become the golden word in the organisation of all modern industries and no less with the NHS, with the recent introduction of general managers.

Management involves the organisation of finances, resources and personnel, for maximum efficiency of the limited resources and to effect the best delivery of care. It relies upon good communication up and down the hierarchy of line managers, from the chief at the DHSS controlling all the resources, down to the people at the grass roots who deliver the service to the consumer.

At different levels of responsibility, staff have variable control over a defined area of administration. In the pyramid structure of nursing, each is accountable to the person in the level above, while supervising the person below.

Management is not a term which nurses find necessarily endearing, nor one with which they are totally at ease, something that may be regarded as unaffecting their particular role. Yet the sister is a manager of her ward, deciding on stock control—ordering of stores, staffing levels—making the off-duty rota, delivery of service—allocation of patients to nurses.

To overcome the mental block that nurses often have about management, learners are introduced to the idea of management skills and how these relate to their role when they become trained nurses. They are involved in problem-solving exercises to do with staff allocation and ward management and are given the opportunity to try running the ward for a day, with a practical assessment on this topic.

Sisters may be offered a first-line management course, usually held at a college, which is often related to management in industry and has little relevance to the health service.

The RCN runs a modular course on management, for nurses who are able to be seconded, which is geared to those at a higher level of management. The more senior nurses are entitled to a course in middle or senior management, looking at topics such as budgeting, recruitment, labour relations, disciplinary procedure, manpower planning and monitoring service.

Nurses in higher managerial positions are expected to liaise with their opposite number in other health service disciplines, with doctors, administrators, finance officers and physiotherapists, in order to give effective team management.

Though nurses may shy away from management, it is important that they hold tight to the reins, lest they find someone else 'managing' the nursing services.

Research

It was strongly recommended in the Briggs Report that nursing should be a research-based profession. With the greater number of university departments for nursing and graduate nurses keen to extend their skills, there has been a notable increase in the research projects on the nursing profession and its practice. Although only a few nurses are directly conducting research, many are involved in projects incidental to their work.

Nurses in basic and post-basic training are introduced to research appreciation, while many courses have been developed for interested trained nurses.

So, how can research in nursing benefit the profession? A gradual build-up of a fund of knowledge will provide the most effective delivery of health care. In one enquiry, for example, it was found that there were around 80 different ways of treating pressure areas and sores—all hit and miss, trial and error, empirical methods, with no rationale or evaluation of their effectiveness.

For research findings to be of any value, they must be disseminated to reach people at the grass roots, if the outcome is to be applied where it is most needed. These findings are frequently reported in the national nursing magazines, available for every practising nurse to read and make use of.

One of the most tangible and useful products has been the *Manual of Clinical Nursing Policies and Procedures* (see page 135), a renovation of the practical work book, based on sound research principles, rather than a 'we've always done it this way' textbook.

There are now several research nursing units in the United Kingdom, and a variety of sources which will fund nurses wanting to undertake a project; the DHSS, in particular, is keen to endorse research into nursing.

There are four main areas where research methods can be successfully and profitably applied, demonstrated here with examples of projects that have been undertaken.

- nursing practice—the effective implementation of the nursing process; how to assess which patients are at risk from pressure sores; how patients perceive pain.

- nursing management—studies on manpower levels; recruitment and wastage; absenteeism among staff; the role of the ward sister.
- nurse education—what makes a suitable clinical learning environment; validation of examination and assessment techniques; career movements of nurses.
- specialist areas of care—primary health care, the role of the district nurse, health visiting practice; intensive care, communication with the unconscious patient; psychiatry, role of the community psychiatric nurse, evaluation of token economy programmes; paediatrics, preparing children for hospitalisation.

Research goes hand in hand with professionalism in nursing and provides the clout of credibility as a scientific discipline. It must form the basis of sound nursing practice and the development of excellence in nursing care. Nurses must be able to measure the effectiveness of the outcome of their actions when giving care to patients.

These days, it is inexcusable for nursing not to be based upon researched and proven information if it is available.

Ethics

Ethics can be described as doing what you 'ought' to do, instead of what you 'want' to do or are coerced into doing. It involves a sense of duty, a sense of moral rightness, based upon acceptable behaviour which comes from within you. This is different from action because you are under obligation to an outside force.

Professional people are expected to adhere to a code of conduct, which is recognised as the way their members behave. Certainly they should not abuse the privileged position of responsibility they have with clients.

So, for example, a woman would expect to feel safe to be undressed in front of a doctor without fear of sexual interference. In other circumstances, outside the professional/client relationship, the situation might be different.

Patients would expect nurses to treat their person and their property with respect while they are under anaesthetic, in a coma or demented. It would be unethical to use bribery to mete out attentions or persuade a patient to alter his will in your favour, when people are dependent on your care.

It is part of professional etiquette and courtesy that nurses resist from favouritism among patients, from being rude or short tempered, that they are loyal to colleagues and always respect confidences within their professional practice.

Our society is encountering an increasing number of dilemmas, as medicine forges further and further past the frontiers controlling birth, life and death. Indeed, by definition, a dilemma is the choice between two unacceptable equals, so even the final resolution will, to some degree, be unsatisfactory and there are rarely any easy, clearcut answers.

For example, someone may consider it terrible to allow a severely handicapped baby to die naturally, whereas another may find it equally awful to subject such an infant to heroic repetitive surgery, that will still only result in a half-life of extreme dependence. It may be unacceptable to use the human embryo for experimental and research purposes, yet equally traumatic to deny research into those crippling inherited diseases that might be avoided.

At the crux of these issues is usually quality versus quantity of existence or the sanctity of life itself, which may be the overriding consideration. When a decision has to be made, people may be directed by their conscience, by religious doctrine, or by a sheer gut reaction.

Medicine now has at its disposal a multitude of lifesaving and life-support facilities and, in many respects, has become the victim of its own success. Doctors may have to justify why they *do not* use treatments available, but even Hippocrates dictated that medicine 'should not strive to keep [someone] officiously alive'.

So the frail, aged person who might in the past have died peacefully from an intercurrent infection, is now rescued from the jaws of death on repeated occasions and may linger on. Pneumonia used to be called the 'old man's friend'—or was it, perhaps, 'the doctor's friend'?!

Congenitally deformed babies, who might have been expected to die from cardiac, neurological or bowel disorders, may now be offered corrective surgery.

Is it tantamount to murder to withhold drugs, surgery, a kidney machine, life support, or an organ transplant? Where does it end and how are the limited resources meted out? A distinction has to be made between 'killing' and 'letting die'. And what is our stand over suicidal patients? One dilemma often leads to another.

Who decides to mobilise resources? Who decides to turn off the machine? Who makes the decision to operate or leave well alone? Should it be left solely to the doctors, for even they vary in their opinions? Should parents have a say, when it is they who will shoulder the burden of caring for their handicapped child? In reality it is usually a joint decision after counselling.

Then again, a married daughter struggling to care for an elderly, demented mother may be keen to hasten along her inheritance, if she were left to decide! Indeed, this poses another question, when should the law intervene to protect the civil liberties of an individual, especially when he may be unable to represent himself, as in the case of the fetus, the patient with severe handicap, dementia, or in a coma?

Obviously the most contentious focal point of all these issues is the possibility of abuse, which would endanger the lives of people who might be considered expendable, especially as regards curtailing or prolonging life. The problem is always when to draw the line, having embarked upon one avenue of action.

Certainly the reader will be familiar with the many areas of conflict which have recently been the subject of heated and emotional debate: embryo experimentation; surrogate motherhood; abortion; resuscitation to extremes; extensive life-support and the criterion of brain death; euthanasia.

In her practical work, the nurse may be faced with a variety of ethical dilemmas. The prescribing of high doses of painkilling drugs for terminal patients may either be successfully alleviating nasty symptoms, or it may be hastening their death.

The nurse may be asked not to administer nourishing feeds to a handicapped baby or to withhold antibiotic drugs. Although the doctor prescribes, it is the nurse who administers to the patient.

Many nurses find it difficult to accept that resuscitation is routine in hospital (unless otherwise specifically stated). They feel repugnance at extreme measures of resuscitation, in apparently hopeless situations, so patients are not allowed to die in dignity. 'No one dies in hospital any more, they are failed resuscitation cases.'

The nurse must act within her conscience, yet she must also be careful to act within the law. No matter how sympathetic she may feel towards euthanasia, it would be illegal for her to assist a patient to his death, likewise to procure an abortion or to acquire drugs for illicit purposes. The Abortion Act carries a conscience clause which allows practitioners to refuse to carry out or assist with the termination of pregnancy.

A nurse is not permitted to refrain from resuscitation—if she were at hand at the point of death—but she could suggest at a team meeting that a certain patient is not a suitable candidate for resuscitation, or has specifically asked not to be subjected to this measure.

If a nurse is ever in doubt she must refer the matter to her senior manager, or she can ask the RCN, who advise on ethical and legal issues in practice.

In general the nurse can be guided by the ethical code stated by the International Council of Nurses in 1973, based upon the four principles of nursing:

- to promote health
- to prevent illness
- to restore health
- to alleviate suffering

within a framework which respects all human life, promotes the dignity and rights of all patients, regardless of age, creed, colour, sex, race, social status or political persuasion.

Reference and refresher reading

Baly M. E. (1984). *Professional Responsibility*. Chichester: John Wiley and Sons Ltd.

Booth J. A. (1983). *Handbook of Investigations*. London: Harper and Row. An excellent update on information about current investigations, with a patient teaching input.

Calnan J. (1984). *Coping with Research*. London: Heinemann Medical Books.

Hunt J. M., Marks-Maran D. J. (1983). *Nursing Care Plans—The Nursing Process at Work*. Chichester: John Wiley and Sons.

Roper N., Logan W., Tierney A. (1980). *The Elements of Nursing*. Edinburgh: Churchill Livingstone. A textbook on nursing based upon a nursing model of care and the problem-solving approach.

The Royal Marsden Hospital (1984). *Manual of Clinical Nursing Policies and Procedures*. London: Harper and Row. The definitive work on clinical procedures, based on sound research findings.

Wilson-Barnett J. (ed.) (1983). *Nursing Research—Ten Studies in Patient Care*. Chichester: John Wiley and Sons.

Young A. P,. (1981). *Legal Problems in Nursing Practice*. London: Harper and Row.

A textbook about the legal side of nursing, written for practising nurses by a nurse tutor.

8

Clinical Developments

The returning nurse will encounter a variety of modern clinical developments and innovations. How many are actually new to her will depend upon her length of absence and the area in which she is currently employed. It is not within the scope of this book to attempt to document and detail *all* the new changes in procedure and commodities that are available in all spheres of nursing. Suffice it to say that current practice has an obligation to keep pace with all developments related to patient care.

New technology

The wealth of advanced knowledge has been harnessed to produce an unprecedented assortment of fascinating wares, resulting in significant changes on the face of modern health care. Although too numerous to mention, a few examples may demonstrate the enormous contribution made by science to medicine and nursing. The use of superior and versatile modern materials have made revolutionary impacts in certain areas.

Biochemical developments have resulted in non-adherent dressings, transparent dressings and impregnated bandages to facilitate wound healing. The complete daily nutritional requirements may be administered via a continuous nasogastric feed or via intravenous infusion, known as total parenteral nutrition (TPN).

Biophysics has lent its expertise to develop laser therapy, refined radiotherapy and fibroptic endoscopy, a flexible tube with reflected light to permit viewing of the body cavities. Interferential therapy will stimulate local circulation, to promote healing and relieve pain, while transcutaneous nerve stimulation (TNS) is used to relieve chronic pain.

The steam kettle has been superseded by the nebuliser, infusion flow can be monitored by a machine counter, and that old problem of deep vein thrombosis (DVT) can be minimised by using graduated compression, antiembolic stockings. Peritoneal dialysis for chronic renal failure, once a lengthy procedure in hospital, can be performed while the patient goes about his daily life, with continuous ambulatory peritoneal dialysis (CAPD).

Precision instruments and lenses facilitate the most intricate microsurgical techniques to reunite ruptured nerves and blood vessels, or correct eye defects. Fibreglass incorporated into a bandage can, when moistened, be modelled into a very strong, highly supportive limb cast, vastly superior to plaster of Paris. Thermoplastic materials, when heated, can be moulded to provide strong, lightweight corsets and splints. Biocompatible metals are successfully implanted as joint prostheses, and are commonly used as the definitive treatment of osteoarthritis. Metals can be fashioned as replicas of diseased bone, which will be accepted by the body, in preference to the trauma of amputation of a limb due to bone neoplasm.

Although the thought of new products and techniques may be daunting to the returning nurse, she should appreciate that these refinements are for the benefit of patients, and many ultimately do aid the nurse in her work. It is to be hoped that significant changes will be demonstrated on a back-to-nursing or orientation course, giving opportunity for returning nurses to handle new equipment.

Anyone introduced to a new area of employment will be taught the tasks and skills relevant to that specialty, and would be expected to take a reasonable time to become acquainted with the new work. This would apply equally to a currently employed nurse who crosses over to a new area of work or one returning to the profession.

One nurse returning to paediatrics found much new technical equipment related to her work. She says she 'found good support and training for specialised technical skills—from tutors, ward staff and technicians. If one was willing to ask questions and admit fears of inadequacy and ignorance, then careful supervision and teaching was always given.' She concludes with the advice, 'Never be afraid to ask'.

In this chapter the aim has been to include those important changes which may be encountered in the general daily routine of the nurse within any area of care.

Central sterile supply department (CSSD), dressings and disposables

The very distinct and resounding impression gained by those

returning to clinical nursing is of an environment with 'disposable everything'! For those used to the impecunious days of rationed stores in locked cupboards, issued by stringent sisters preaching economy, the situation of today seems a rash contrast with its lavish and plentiful supply of prepackaged goods.

Gone are the dressing drums and cheetle forceps, the night nurses preparing swabs, to such an extent that it is a rarity even to find a sterilising unit on a ward.

Every nurse with a clinical role, working either in hospital or the community, has access to the district *central sterile supply department* or *unit* (CSSD or CSSU). Specialist staff are concerned with the control of cross-infection and infection hazards within the district and there is usually an *infection control sister* (ICS).

A variety of packs are prepared to particular specification to suit many needs, such as simple dressings, suturing, lumbar puncture, mid-stream urine specimen or thoracotomy. From the smallest job in accident and emergency departments to the largest job in a critical emergency, a pack containing all the necessary items is available to each ward and department.

Packs contain a tray, galley pot and forceps, all of which are ostensibly disposable, but can be recycled through CSSD to be used several times over. Items are wrapped in a paper or linen sheet, which doubles as a sterile field when opened out. The whole pack is assembled in a bag made of special paper which is impervious to microbes, provided it remains dry and intact, thus having a reasonable shelf life.

The CSSD operates a top-up service on a daily basis, to fill the racks with replacement packs and take away used items for resterilisation.

Commercial companies are increasingly providing disposable sterile packages and individually wrapped items, usually sterilised by gamma ray irradiation. The outer wrapping carries a detailed list of contents and an explanation of how the item is to be used.

Disposable forceps made of plastic or metal have not proved popular, as they are difficult to manipulate. Plastic gloves tend to be preferred when doing extensive dressings, such as for burns or traumatic injuries, rather than struggling with fiddly forceps.

Paper masks are not considered effective or necessary and have largely been discontinued for general ward procedures.

Multidose lotion bottles can become a breeding ground for

microbes and a source of cross-infection as they pass from trolley to trolley, from patient to patient. Solutions are now generally dispensed in commercially prepared individual dose sachets.

The disposal of dangerous sharp items poses a considerable health hazard to nurses and porters, who may inadvertently receive a skin puncture or laceration while transporting rubbish bags. 'Sharps' include injection needles, infusion needles, stitch cutters and used glass ampoules, which must be carefully deposited in a safe 'sharps' impenetrable container.

The nurse will find an enviable assortment of disposable items ready for her use in every situation. Sometimes these can be safely reused in the interest of economy, such as plastic draw-sheets or crêpe bandages that can be disinfected between patients. A diabetic patient may reuse the same needle and syringe, and a person needing intermittent catheterisation may reuse one catheter on several occasions.

The availability of soft plastic has superseded the old red rubber tubing across the full spectrum of nursing care: naso-gastric, urinary, wound drainage, endotracheal, tracheostomy, intrathoracic, suction and intravenous tubing, as well as stoma and urine-collecting bags. Previous fragile glass items which needed to be cleaned and resterilised have now been replaced by durable plastic with graduated markings, among them syringes, intravenous fluid bottles, burettes and the lumbar puncture manometer.

Nurses no longer wear linen aprons with the national uniform but don disposable thin plastic aprons for individual nursing procedures.

A milk kitchen is needed nowadays only for preparation of special formulas or expressed breast milk (EBM), as all other regular baby feeds are delivered in prepackaged, sterile, one-feed bottles, be it water, dextrose or baby milk.

Urine testing is universally performed with the reagent-impregnated dipstrips or tablets sensitive to changes and abnormalities in a specimen.

From a vast catalogue of disposables comes: oxygen masks, electrode skin stickers, theatre overshoes and masks, nappies, nurses' paper caps and bedpans.

The 'use once and destroy' concept may at first sight seem extravagant but there are two very distinct advantages. Goods reach the patient with guaranteed sterility, which minimises the possibility of cross-infection at source. Also, the cleansing and repackaging of instruments, tubing and laundry is labour-intensive and, considering the overriding cost of staff salaries, it is often more cost-effective to buy in one-off disposable items.

Nurses are no longer required to learn in parrot fashion lists of trays and trolleys, although they are expected to know the contents of packs and the extra items needed to carry out clinical procedures. Returning nurses would be instructed in the methods related to aseptic techniques which involve the use of sterile packs.

Ward equipment

There is a wide selection of equipment on the market designed to ease the work of the nurse, increase patient comfort and improve safe handling for both parties. The availability of this equipment is subject to local variation, as many of the larger items do involve a substantial financial commitment. However, this initial capital outlay proves to be a sensible investment, with obvious benefits to patient care, and the fact that these items have a long working life.

With the notable prevalence of back injury amongst nurses, there has been a greater inclination for authorities to adopt the use of hoists. Once the staff have gained confidence in using hoists, they are enthusiastically accepted by nurses and patients alike. They quickly become popular and valued ward accessories, providing a safe and effective way of lifting, moving and bathing heavy and dependent patients.

In areas such as a ward bathroom, physiotherapy department or in a disabled person's bedroom at home, an electrically operated hoist may be fixed to the ceiling, to allow the patient to manoeuvre himself up, down and along using pulley cords.

Bathroom equipment

A mobile mechanical hoist has a more general use within a ward and can be operated by one nurse with the minimum effort, thereby obviating the risk of back injury. The Mecanaids Ambulift, shown in Figure 8.1, is the most commonly used in hospitals; the patient sits comfortably and securely, able to be wheeled to the bath, lowered into the water, washed and dried, while remaining well-supported on the seat.

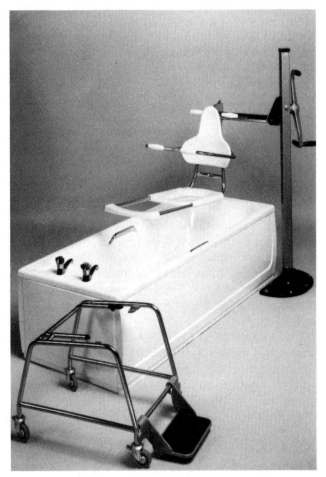

Fig. 8.1   Mecanaids fixed-base bathing hoist.

This versatile piece of equipment comes with modifications, either to make into a toilet chair or to have a commode-pan attachment, or the hoist can be a static fixture in a bathroom. An electronic scale attachment enables nurses to weigh patients quickly and accurately without manual lifting.

Other versions have sling attachments, one for sitting upright (Figure 8.2) one for lying horizontal, particularly useful for frail or emaciated patients or those with pressure sores, all of whom may find a conventional firm chair uncomfortable.

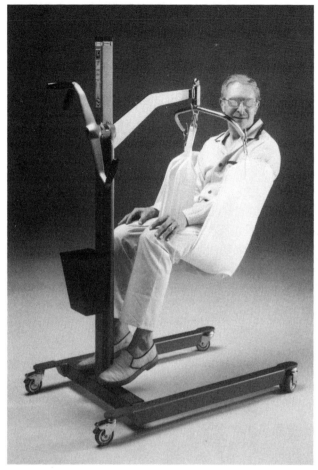

Fig. 8.2 Mecanaids Ambulift with sling attachment.

Various designs for modern baths can assist dependent or disabled patients to enjoy a normal bath and protect nurses from back strain.

An upright bath, built like an open-top cabinet with watertight sealable sides, enables a patient to sit down and his body to be immersed in water.

Variable-height baths have a double benefit. The patient has ease of access when the bath is lowered, while the nurse, rather than continually stooping, can wash her patient at the more con-

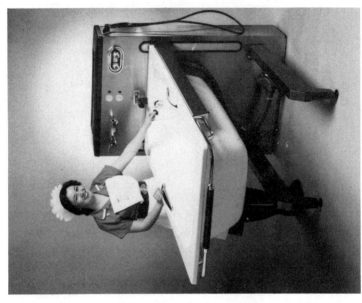

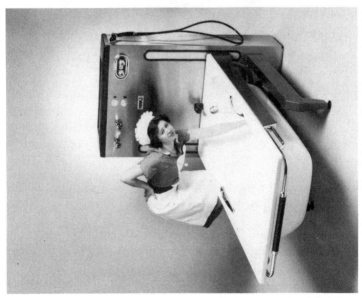

Fig. 8.3A and B   Mecanaids Hi-Lo bath with the variable height facility.

venient higher level. Figure 8.3 (A and B) demonstrates the Hi-Lo bath.

Beds and bedding

Hospital beds generally have the variable-height facility; the Kings Fund bed, operated manually to lower the bed or tilt either end, is useful in a variety of situations.

The perennial problem of pressure sores is as great a menace today as ever it was. Several new innovations have been designed to reduce the incidence of sores in vulnerable patients, to promote the opportunity to heal established sores, and to provide comfort for those confined to bed.

The low air loss bed works on the hovercraft principle, to provide even distribution of body weight and relieve pressure from dependent parts. A Stryker frame facilitates frequent, easy turning by a single nurse, to alternate pressure from both front and back of the patient.

A net suspension bed provides pressureless support with air circulation and enables simple, effortless turning of the occupant by one nurse. The Mecabed, shown in Figure 8.4, fits over any

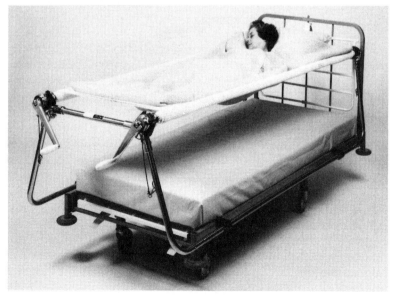

Fig. 8.4   The Mecabed net suspension bed by Mecanaids.

type of bed. The patient is cocooned in the bedding and cradled in the net support which is firmly suspended between two longitudinal poles.

Various different mattresses, filled either with water, gel, beads or foam, are available to reduce or redistribute pressure around the body. The ripple mattress comprises cells of air, alternating to give varying areas of inflation and deflation.

Other smaller aids are found in general use, such as supportive foam padding, sorbo rings and articles made of sheepskin, all aimed at reducing the likelihood of pressure sores developing.

Returning nurses would have full instruction in the handling of any equipment that they will be expected to use in the course of their work, and this also applies to any of the sophisticated electrical items employed in modern patient care.

SI units

With the global expansion of technological, scientific and medical advances, it became necessary to determine international standards of measurement. A system was required that would be universally recognisable, to permit ready exchange of valuable information throughout the world.

The Système International d'Unités, commonly known as SI units, was formally adopted in British hospitals in 1975. The conversion is gradually being accepted as personnel become acquainted with the new measurements, and it is now a legal requirement in the United Kingdom for drugs to be prescribed and dispensed in SI units.

The SI system is based upon the former metric system, so there will be some terms with which nurses are already familiar in everyday life, such as gram (g) for food, litre (l) for fluids and metre (m) for length of material and clothes sizing.

When decimal currency was introduced, the advice was to 'think decimal' and work within the new system, rather than trying to convert and compare with the old money. So it should be when you first encounter SI units—'think SI'. Become familiar with the new measurements as you are required to use them in your working life and adjust to arithmetic within the system.

There are seven basic units of measurement of practical relevance to the nurse. These are shown in Table 8.1.

Table 8.1 SI units and how they are written

Unit	Written
Length—metre	m
Mass—kilogram	kg
Volume—litre	l
Energy—joule	J
Pressure—pascal	Pa
Amount of substance—mole	mol
Temperature—degree Celsius	°C

Units become larger or smaller in ten-fold graduations, with each denomination having a standard prefix.

For example, using the basic unit of length, the metre: as it gets bigger,

> 10 units is a decametre, written dam
> 100 units is a hectometre, written hm
> 1000 units is a kilometre, written km

as it gets smaller,

> 0.1 is a decimetre, written dm
> 0.01 is a centimetre, written cm
> 0.001 is a millimetre, written mm
> 0.000 001 is a micrometre, written μm

Likewise, the nurse will commonly work with the kilogram (kg) which is 1000 grams (g), and the milligram (mg), which is 1000th of a gram. The kilogram is roughly equivalent to 2 lb, so one might bear in mind a bag of sugar when considering weight.

Patients are now routinely weighed in kilograms, including babies in the maternity unit and infant clinics. However, for some time yet, until the youth of today is completely oriented to SI units, the public will still expect to hear weights expressed in stones, pounds and ounces. The nurse can be reassured that in the vicinity of every weighing scale she will find a direct conversion chart that requires no calculations.

The joule (J) is gradually replacing the calorie as the measurement unit of heat, but is still not common parlance to the diet-conscious public, who continue to 'count calories'.

One noticeable change for returning nurses is in biochemical values that are expressed in SI units and may look strange at first. It is vital that you blot out and forget the old values you once knew and become familiar with the new normal values, in order that you can recognise abnormal variations. For example: haemoglobin—the normal range for an adult is expressed as 12–18 g/dl; plasma urea—the normal range for an adult is 2.5–6.6 mmol/l.

Pascal (Pa), the measurement of pressure, has not yet been widely adopted in practice, but in the future should be used when estimating blood pressure. So a systolic blood pressure of 150 mmHg would read 20 kPa in SI measurements.

Temperature is consistently measured in SI in all areas of nursing, using the degree Celsius (often mistakenly called Centigrade). The nurse must become fully conversant with the Celsius scale and develop a working understanding of both normal ranges and abnormal variations encountered in patient care (Figure 8.5; Table 8.2). To convert degrees F to degrees C, subtract 32 then multiply by ⅝. To convert degrees C into degrees F, multiply by ⅝ and add 32.

Blood for transfusion and allied substances is no longer measured in pints, but prepared in 'units', each unit containing 500 ml of fluid. So a patient may have a blood sample taken to cross-match three units of blood for use during surgery.

CLINICAL THERMOMETERS

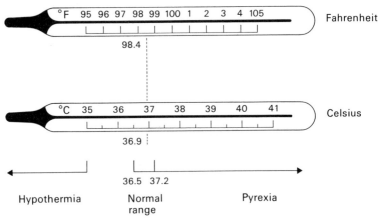

Fig. 8.5   The Celsius and Fahrenheit temperature scales.

Table 8.2 Normal and abnormal temperature ranges

Freezing point of water	0 °C
Boiling point of water	100 °C
Range of normal temperature	36.5–37.2 °C (average = 36.9 °C)
Hypothermia	below 35 °C
Pyrexia	above 37.2 °C

The nurse will also find the 24-hour clock in more prevalent use: for example, 2 pm is 14.00 hours and 10 pm is 22.00 hours.

In conclusion, SI units, because of the decimal arithmetic, are much easier to use when working out measurements (see reference and refresher reading, page 159). *However, extreme caution must be taken not to be confused by the number of 0s involved and to ensure correct placing of the decimal point, especially when calculating paediatric drug doses.*

Drugs

One of the greatest anxieties facing the returning nurse, after even the briefest absence, is the dread of being out of date with drugs in current use. It is an understandable concern for the trained nurse, who is responsible for the safe administration of drugs and the supervision of patients receiving them. There appear to be so many to master all at one go, with difficult names, varied actions and side-effects, while learners and patients enquire about them.

Let us commence by being utterly realistic about this topic. Nobody can master the facts pertaining to all the many drugs on the market, nor, indeed, is anyone expected to. Rest assured that it is virtually impossible to keep abreast of the volatile changes on the drugs scene—unless you have a photographic memory or an all-consuming passion for pharmacology! It is a minefield of rapidly changing names, as competitors jostle to claim their stake in the drugs market.

So always keep the drugs situation in perspective.

You can reasonably be expected to become familiar with the medications that you will be using in day-to-day work in your area of allocation. These you should know well, especially side-effects and toxic effects to be aware of, as well as any specific instructions regarding administration, such as with meals, before meals, in the morning, at night, or any concurrent foods and drugs to be avoided. Make an effort to learn the generic or phar-macological names alongside brand names, as doctors are now being urged to prescribe the cheaper BP, non-branded prep-arations, as opposed to the excessively priced proprietary brands supplied by drug companies.

In your induction period, when you know where you will be working, ask the ward sister to give you a list of the drugs com-monly used in the ward. Take it away and do your homework.

Books about drugs in the 'materia medica' style go out of date as fast as they are printed, and books from your student days will be of limited help. However, there are several good general books available, which are useful because they discuss the principles behind groups of drugs, such as antibiotics, steroids, tranquil-lisers etc. They give sound information on basic pharmacological use and action, without getting bogged down with too many specific drugs, so would be a useful refresher aid for the returning nurse.

The reference guides produced for doctors are reproduced monthly, which gives some indication of the fluidity of the drug market! These guides are the simplest, most effective way of researching individual drugs, as they document relevant infor-mation in an easily presented fashion.

You should have at hand a current *MIMS* (*Monthly Index of Medical Specialties*). One is ideally available for reference in every clinical situation and you may find that the pharmacist will let you have your own copy of a recent 'old' one.

Another similar guide for reference is the *BNF* (*British National Formulary*), which is widely available and can be obtained through a bookseller.

Junior nurses would be interested in these two useful guides, so do make their inquiries into a learning exercise for you both. They won't expect you to be a walking pharmacopoeia but will appreciate it if you take the trouble to find out with them.

Once you start delving into pharmacology, you will find many types of medication that you recognise of old, masquerading behind a variety of fancy brand names. You will also be pleasantly surprised to find a considerable hard core of drugs that have stood the time for efficiency, have retained popularity and continue to be prescribed. You will be familiar with aspirin, paracetamol, codeine, frusemide, digoxin, heparin, pethidine and many, many more.

Barbiturate drugs have fallen out of favour because of their addictive nature, whereas other safer sedatives have taken their place. Antiarthritic drugs, the group known as NSAIDs or non-steroidal anti-inflammatory drugs, are constantly being manufactured, while some have been discredited by causing adverse reactions. Antibiotics tend to be changed quite frequently, once bacteria develop a resistance to established drugs.

Exciting progress is being made with cytotoxic drugs, used to combat malignant conditions. Drugs which suppress the immune system have grown apace to facilitate organ transplantation, and to prevent rejection of the donor organ, and these have contributed to the current level of success in this field.

Paediatric medication is usually packaged in a pleasant-tasting liquid suspension, which makes the administration of oral drugs a painless procedure for children—and their mothers and nurses. *However, extreme care must always be taken over the precise calculation of paediatric doses given by any route.*

Extra care should also be taken when prescribing for the elderly, as they may be incapable of dealing with complicated regimes involving a wide variety of drugs and instructions—two pink in the morning, one blue at lunchtime, 5 ml of syrup morning and night, half a beige pill in the evening and one white one before resting, for example!

It is also necessary to be aware of the decreased tolerance of drugs in the elderly and the toxic effects of accumulated doses due to inadequate clearance by the body. Yet another danger is overmedication from various sources: general practitioner, hospital doctor, over-the-counter preparations, persisting with discontinued prescriptions, so that any beneficial effects are lost as drugs counteract one another. It may also result in drug-induced complications, resulting in hospitalisation for reassessment of the patient's drug regime.

The Misuse of Drugs Act (1971)

The Misuse of Drugs Act (1971) is concerned with those drugs likely to cause addiction or dependence, such as pethidine, methadone, papaveretum (Omnopon), morphine, diamorphine (heroin). The specific procedures related to these 'controlled drugs' (CDA) vary little from those for the previous 'dangerous drugs' (DDA).

- containers are labelled CDA
- containers are locked in a specific CDA wall cupboard
- CDA keys are held by a trained nurse
- CDA drugs are ordered in a special book and signed for on receipt
- CDA drugs and administration details are checked by two nurses, one of whom must be registered or of senior enrolled status (this depends on local policy).
- when giving a CDA there is rigid checking of prescription details; patient's identity, the date, drug and dose, route, time of administration, doctor's signature; details are recorded on the individual drug sheet, on the Kardex, as well as in the CDA record book which is signed by both nurses.

Drugs governed by legislation in Schedule I of the Poisons List (such as barbiturates, atropine and digoxin) and Schedule IV (such as diazepam and chloral hydrate) are potentially harmful and subject to abuse. These are also locked away, and have to be stored separately and checked at each administration against the patient's prescription and the stock balance.

The recently adopted simplified method of insulin preparation is an undeniable blessing, compared to the old method requiring calculation. Insulin now comes in U100 strength, to be given with a U100 syringe, which is 1 ml divided into 100 parts or 0.5 ml divided into 50 parts. So if 10 units of U100 insulin are prescribed, then 10 divisions are given measured on a U100 syringe. This is so much more straightforward than the confusion from multiplying or dividing with varied strengths of old insulin.

Computers

In common with virtually every other aspect of the modern world, there is an increasing interest in the application of computer technology to medical and nursing practice and health administration. With the promise of much more to come in this rapidly developing area, there is a nursing specialist group within the British Computer Society, to keep the profession abreast of changes.

Certainly any study days or courses on computer literacy are eagerly seized and frequently oversubscribed by nurses keen to acquaint themselves with these exciting developments. At present, those most proficient with computers are young nurses, who have recently been involved with computer studies at school, and older nurses, whose teenage children have brought the idea into the home with their personal computer. However, any nurse who is expected to use a computer in the course of her work must be reassured that she would be adequately prepared in computer literacy.

This is an area of rapid expansion, although of variable application within different health authorities, hospitals and schools of nursing, depending on their enlightenment and financial situation. No book could hope to keep pace with the computer explosion, so what follows is a resumé of the major ways in which computers are being applied to benefit contemporary health care.

Information storage and retrieval

- *at ward level*   documentation of patient care plans, similar to the Kardex, medical notes with investigation results and prescriptions.
- *administration*   documentation of patient complement, bed state, forward planning for admission and discharge, waiting list; district personnel records system, recruitment, staff establishment, salary, leave dates, sickness, appraisal.
- *training school*   record of learners past and present, allocation, training programme, holidays, sick leave, ward assessments.
- *community*   documentation of patients on general practitioners list, monitoring health changes, formulating 'at risk' register, call back for routine screening list, for instance cervical cytology and infant immunisation programme, allocation of staff according to workload and travel.

Used in any of these areas, a computer can reduce the amount of paperwork and confine information to one central source. Care must be taken that personal information is not divulged or abused by allowing unauthorised access, to cause a breach in confidence. However, statistical analysis gives a helpful guide to

assist both manpower and service planning in relation to anticipated patient needs.

Education

- Computer-assisted learning (CAL), see page 195.
- Marking of multiple-choice question papers.

Clinical application

- Computerised monitoring and analysis of observations, infusions and pathological specimens
- Appliances to assist the disabled with mobility and com-munication (Figure 8.6).
- Computer-assisted tomography (CAT).

Conventional X-rays, which have been in use for almost a cen-tury, are ideal for showing bone and calcium deposits and air. Any soft tissue must be demonstrated by use of a radio-opaque contrast dye, such as barium. In either event, the picture pro-duced is flat and two-dimensional, giving no indication of depth.

A tomogram takes a series of pictures, like slices of a loaf, to il-lustrate structures three-dimensionally, and these have been very useful, for example, to give the precise location of a lesion in the lung.

Computer-assisted tomography (CAT), using a sophisticated piece of machinery generally known as a 'scanner', has revolu-tionised diagnostic imaging. By taking multiple, low-powered X-ray beams across the body or head, a picture is built up from the 'slices' by the computer, to give a clear illustration of a cross-section. It is safe, simple and highly effective, and can diagnose abnormalities even before they are large enough to cause clinical problems. Unfortunately the cost of a machine to buy, house and operate is enormous, so scanners have become the object of many worthwhile charity collections over recent years.

Cardiopulmonary resuscitation (CPR)

When the action of the heart fails and it ceases to beat, this is known as cardiac arrest, and is immediately followed by ces-sation of breathing, or respiratory arrest. These combined quickly lead to circulatory collapse and death.

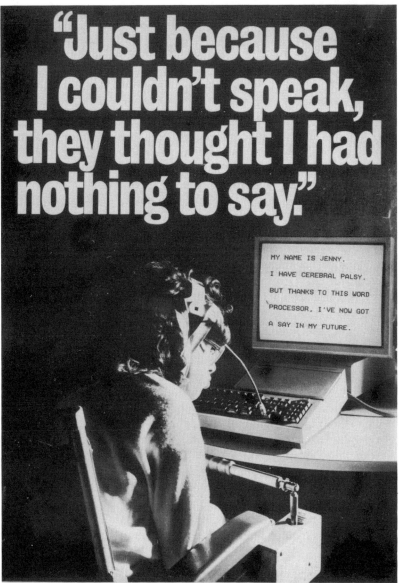

Fig. 8.6 Computers can help the disabled to communicate.
(Poster reproduced by kind permission of The Spastics Society.)

With prompt and effective management of cardiopulmonary resuscitation (CPR) (see Figure 8.7), it may be possible to reverse this process and restore the circulation. Speed of commencement and efficiency in method are both crucial to the successful outcome of CPR, as only four minutes are left in which to begin action, beyond which time there may be irreversible brain damage due to anoxia.

CPR is performed universally in the first aid situation, either to revive a patient or sustain him in a reasonable condition until medical assistance can be sought. The use of CPR is widely taught to adult groups and teenagers, as a viable measure to be undertaken by any member of the public in a crisis.

The management of CPR in a hospital obviously extends beyond these immediate measures, to make use of a well-trained team of personnel and all the sophisticated equipment and drugs available. An on-call team would comprise an anaesthetist, several doctors, a senior nurse, possibly an anaesthetic nurse, and the porter who brings the resuscitation trolley packed with all the necessary items for CPR. A team is summoned by a crash call, which is the emergency internal telephone number that must be made familiar to all staff members to use as their initial response.

If handled well, CPR can prove to be a highly successful procedure and is certainly always worth a try. Many people walking around today have cause to be grateful to someone who made the correct response and initiated action speedily. In hospital, it is the medical staff who decide on the resuscitation status of each patient, taking account of the person's age, medical condition and prognosis. Those who are not deemed suitable for resuscitation will carry some indication of this, either in their Kardex or on the medical notes, and should be known by all staff.

Obviously the most likely cause of cardiac arrest is a myocardial infarction of a severe degree, but CPR is also applicable after electrocution, drowning, asphyxia, suffocation, drug overdose and severe shock or haemorrhage following surgical catastrophe or injury.

The correct administration of CPR is a skill of paramount importance for every nurse to master, so it is taught most thoroughly to both new entrants and returning nurses, with periodic revision thereafter. Theoretical instruction of the principles is followed by practical demonstration on a dummy, which has inflatable lungs and a palpable pulse. Plenty of opportunity is given for individual practice in this first aid technique. Those nurses who work in accident and emergency departments and intensive care units will have the greatest involvement with CPR on a regular basis.

Assessment of the patient in need of CPR is shown by the CPR criteria: the *6 Cs.*

- collapse
- consciousness lost
- carotid pulse absent
- cessation of breathing
- colour, ashen and/or cyanosis
- circumference of pupils dilated.

The underlying principles of CPR are based upon A B C
   A = airway   B = breathing   C = circulation

Immediate action of CPR

Put the patient on a flat, firm surface and loosen necktie/corsets or belt. Stand beside the casualty, or kneel if he is on the ground.

Airway
Clear the *airway*. Remove anything from the mouth that may be causing a possible obstruction to the airway: dentures, food debris, vomit, blood; pull the tongue forward (Figure 8.7A).
Maintain patency of the airway by hyperextending the neck. Place one hand under the neck, another on the forehead and tilt head backwards (Figure 8.7B).

Breathing
Initiate *artificial ventilation* (otherwise called mouth-to-mouth resuscitation or the kiss of life).
Pinch the nose closed. Pull the jaw down to open the mouth (Figure 8.7C). Inhale deeply and cover the casualty's mouth by your mouth, forming an airtight seal, and blow hard.
Glance sideways to observe the rise and fall of the chest to check if the ventilation has been successful (Figure 8.7D).

Circulation
Initial *sternal thump*. Locate the lower end of the sternum and give one short, sharp thump. Check carotid pulse—if not present

then commence *external cardiac massage.* Place one hand on top of the other and, using the heel of the lower hand, apply pressure to the lower half of the sternum. Rock forward, using the weight of your body to depress the breastbone 3–5 cm (Figure 8.7E).

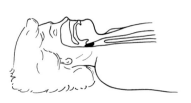

A. Clear airway of blockage

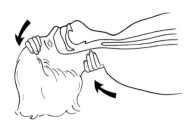

B. Position head to keep airway patent

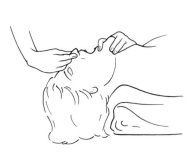

C. Pinch nostrils. Pull jaw down

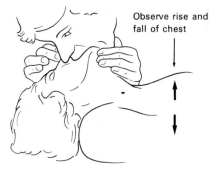

Observe rise and fall of chest

D. Seal mouth by operators mouth. Blow hard

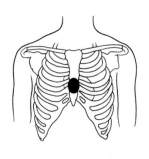

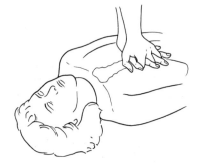

E. External cardiac compression

Fig. 8.7 Cardiopulmonary resuscitation.

If working alone, continue by giving 15 chest compressions, followed by two inflations—this is very tiring and cannot be sustained by one person for very long. When doing the procedure with two operators, one gives five compressions, then stops to allow his partner to give one inflation.

Further action in CPR procedure

When this occurs in hospital, or if the patient is transferred, further measures can be adopted to stabilise the casualty's condition.

Airway
Rubber airway; endotracheal intubation; suction apparatus.

Breathing
Ambubag; oxygen; mechanical ventilation.

Circulation
ECG and oscilloscope; X-ray; defibrillator; intravenous infusion (IVI), cutdown set; urinary catheterisation; reverse metabolic acidosis with intravenous sodium bicarbonate; plus drugs such as adrenaline, calcium chloride, atropine, aminophylline, lignocaine, isoprenaline, frusemide.

Reference and refresher reading

First Aid Manual (1982). St John Ambulance Society. London: Dorling Kindersley.

Parrish P. (1985). *Medicines—A Guide for Everybody*, 5th edn. Harmondsworth: Penguin Books.

MIMS Monthly Index of Medical Specialties. London: Haymarket Publishing Ltd. Monthly.

BNF British National Formulary. London: British Medical Association. A twice-yearly publication.

David J. (1984). *Drug Round Companion*. Oxford: Blackwell Scientific.

Glenn J., McCaugherty D. (1981). *SI Units for Nurses*. London: Harper and Row.
    This book has been written expressly for practising nurses who wish to get to grips with SI units, by providing relevant information on the topic and self-instructional tests.

9

The Profession of Nursing

Professional identity

For a long time, nursing suffered from being seen as a mere backup service to the medical profession, without any specific identity of its own. Nurses were the ones who took orders, carried out the doctors' instructions implicitly and without question, while being in that unique position of giving round-the-clock attention to every patient, on a personal basis.

The potential diversity of the nurse's function in a huge variety of situations makes it particularly difficult to clarify her role. It is equally difficult to make a precise definition of what constitutes the profession of nursing.

It is not easy to give an answer to the question, 'What does a nurse do?'. Think of her function in accident and emergency departments, for instance, compared to a district nurse, or a theatre nurse compared to one working in psychiatric rehabilitation.

Yet there must be a core to each of these roles, something which loosely links all types of nurses, while also differentiating nursing from other health care professionals. Although the work of the physiotherapist and the nurse frequently overlap and each may help the other with patient management, both professionals retain distinct functions within the team.

Probably the best attempt is the classic definition of nursing by Virginia Henderson, which is sufficiently broad to encompass all areas of nursing care.

Nursing is primarily the assisting of the individual (sick or well), in the performance of those activities contributing to health, or its recovery (or to a peaceful death), that he would perform unaided if he had the necessary strength, will or knowledge. It is likewise the unique contribution of nursing to help the individual to be independent of such assistance as soon as possible.

This is represented in diagrammatic form in Figure 9.1.

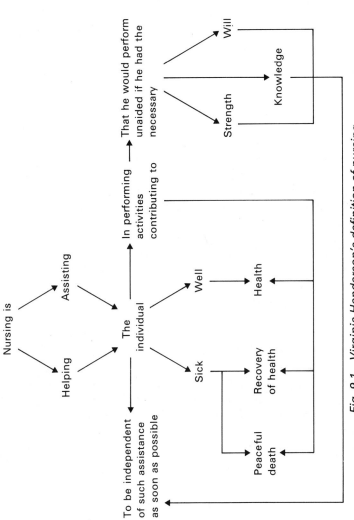

Fig. 9.1 Virginia Henderson's definition of nursing.

Certainly, the introduction of the nursing process went a long way to help clarify the specific function of a nurse within the framework of the caring team. She takes a nursing history and uses that information to devise, implement and evaluate a nursing care plan for each individual patient. The nurse has the ultimate responsibility for decisions in her sphere of function and is accountable for her performance within the boundaries of her role.

Working alongside colleagues in the health care team, the nurse makes an equal contribution to the total management of a patient. A hospital team generally comprises doctor, physiotherapist, social worker, occupational therapist and nurse, while in the community the nurse and health visitor work with the general practitioner and social worker. The nurse is no longer the silent member who hands the X-rays and pours the coffee, she is part of the decision-making process of a multidisciplinary team of professionals.

As individuals, nurses were handicapped by the strong traditional notion of nursing as a pure vocation: the idea of kindly ladies devoted to their work, which was acknowledged to be grim in parts, but who loved their task and were not overly concerned about financial reward. But nurses have to eat and pay for accommodation like every other worker and do deserve more than admiration in the modern world.

Undoubtedly, the women's movement, keen to pursue equal pay and opportunities and to develop career prospects for females, helped to pull nursing free of its historic ideology and to propel it into a profession. Concurrent developments within nursing helped to improve its standing, elevate its status and create the distinct identity that it so badly needed. The academic input and the use of the nursing model of care instead of the medical model were important, as was the introduction of research into nursing practice and management, and degree courses with nursing as a discipline.

With the new era of professionalism, it was seen necessary to educate the general public about the position of nurses in society. Great efforts were made to expound the *image*, in what became known as the Public Image of Nurses Campaign (PINC) (Figure 9.2). This was levelled in particular at the media, who had persisted in depicting stereotyped false images, which were clearly not representative of the real life work of a nurse. Their extremes were defamatory to the profession, and belittling or offensive because of their suggestive nature.

The main targets were the familiar parodies that appear with frequency on our screens and hoardings. The blonde, attractive lithe young student with miniscule skirt revealing suspenders and the obligatory black stockings was either hilarious because she was naive, dumb and clumsy, or blatantly degraded as a willing sex object, a character common to the blue movie.

The large, amply bosomed matron was depicted as a battle-axe, a powerful figure concerned with compliant patients and chastising lesser members of staff who quaked in her presence. Even those who adopted the persona of the dedicated career woman did so at the expense of their femininity, either stripped of all sex appeal or so desperate that she was putty in the hands of

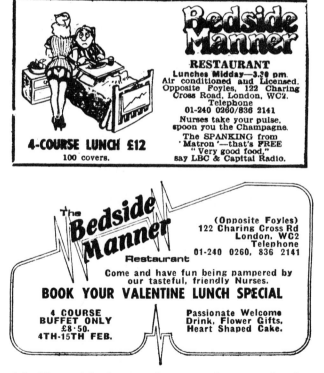

Fig. 9.2 The public image of nurses: the top advertisement appeared in 1983. After the PINC campaign, it was changed to the still objectionable but less offensive advertisement below.

any passing doctor. He, as any hospital romance clearly shows, is handsome, rugged, moody with a tender spot inside, waiting for the right nurse to melt his emotions! Doctors too have suffered from image stereotyping but theirs has been much more flattering and acceptable, because it never questions or challenges their role.

These stereotypes are so ingrained, that rarely do male nurses get a mention, or any of the 'ordinary' nurses beyond the age of 25 who are married with a family and upholding a job of responsibility. However, some of the media documentaries and the soap operas do redress the balance in depicting current nursing life.

It is difficult to believe that anyone who had ever received any nursing care could have held these farfetched images to be true. Nevertheless, it seemed timely to quash the caricatures, get the books straight once and for all, to raise the standard of representation for the profession, so that it would reflect the truth about her role. Some areas of the campaign achieved notable success after pressure from large numbers of nurses.

By making their feelings known, their voices heard and their presence felt, nurses are being urged to 'get *political*' in both senses of the word. They are expected to show an interest in internal politics within the profession and actively participate in changes that affect their work, such as future training plans or development of specialist roles.

Nurses, either collectively or individually, are also encouraged to use their considerable weight through governmental politics, to state their views nationwide. As both employees and consumers of the NHS, they are ideally placed to offer their views and may influence recommendations and decisions about health provision. They can put forward their case regarding such issues as surrogate motherhood, community care for psychiatric patients or legislation about family planning or drug abuse. They can also act as a pressure group for an improved deal for nurses as an occupational group over items like pay and the sale of nurses' homes. There are currently two nurses with a peerage who sit in the House of Lords.

Nurses could have a substantial influence but, as yet, have been unwilling or lacking in confidence to state their opinions firmly in public, as do their medical colleagues. Some specialist groups have organised themselves to make their views known, both to other professionals and to the public, such as the Radical Nurses Group, Association of Radical Midwives and Radical Health Visitors.

As individual citizens, or through corporate representation like the RCN, the nurse's voice must be heard loud and strong. This in turn will reflect well on the profession as a responsible and respectable body of people, whose modern image will be in the public eye.

The clinical nurse specialist

Derived from the professional identity has evolved a new breed of clinical nurse specialist, whose expertise encircles a certain topic of care, such as diabetic management, stoma care, breast care, or continence adviser. She develops her knowledge and skills about the defined subject, which are then delivered across the spectrum of patient administration, allocating her expertise wherever it is needed.

For example, the stoma care specialist will be involved in counselling patients and relatives in both the preoperative and postoperative phase, together with advice and management of the stoma and appliances. Having an autonomous and peripatetic role within the district, she could be found in any of the wards, in the outpatient department or in the community, working alongside those who are giving total care. Indeed, any clinical nurse specialist serves a particularly useful role in bridging the gap between hospital and community, able to maintain important links with patients in her care.

The nurse specialist is an accredited source of information and experience, knowing her subject in great depth and breadth, which she can share with colleagues, patients, relatives and lay groups.

Successive policy-makers have recognised the inestimable value of the trained nurse as the one who plans and delivers care to the patient at the grass roots. It has been a constant matter of concern that keen, competent and experienced clinical nurses may be lured away from the bedside by the incentives of salary and status of higher posts in administration and education. This has been acknowledged as an unsatisfactory arrangement for both the service and the individual nurse, who may prefer to remain in the clinical environment.

So, instead of eroding the clinical role, there has been a concerted effort to strengthen the grade of sister and charge nurse, who have the unique position as leaders of the team directly concerned with patient care. The aim is to develop the clinical career of the nurse, to enable her to become a *clinical practitioner*, on an equal level with teachers and managers.

Non-nursing duties

Having clarified what nurses do, it became necessary to define very specifically what nurses do *not* do. Many tasks, which traditionally fell to the nurse when no one else was available, such as cleaning, damp dusting, washing up and clearing meal trays, became outlawed as non-nursing duties and were allocated to other groups of staff.

Ancillary work is now the total responsibility of the administrator. Ward cleaners, domestic and catering staff come under the aegis of the *hotel services manager* and it is to him that sister refers if she is dissatisfied with the service. To some extent, nurses are sorry to have lost control of ward ancillary staff, because they may also lose the loyalty, goodwill and personal contact with those who should be an integral part of the ward team and provide continuity.

One task which has proved contentious is the supervision of patients' meals. Although the ward domestic will deliver the preordered plated meal and collect the debris, it should be the ultimate responsibility of the nurse to ensure that the patient is actually consuming an adequate diet.

Many of the routine clerical duties can be given to the *ward clerk*, to relieve nursing staff of administrative work such as answering the telephone, arranging appointments, ordering transport, filing forms, preparing notes for doctors' rounds, giving out patients' post, or completing menu forms.

Volunteers, who can provide a useful adjunct to any ward for a variety of tasks, may be allocated and supervised by a *volunteer service coordinator*.

Demographic changes and nurses

Demographic changes within the general society are bound to reflect on the population within nursing, resulting in several marked differences since the last generation.

Sociologists refer to the phenomenon of 'the disappearing spinster'. There is no such thing any longer as the 'maiden aunt' tagging onto the nuclear family and bachelor ladies are no longer called 'spinsters'. If single women have no husband or children, they make a life for themselves by pursuing useful, interesting jobs, developing social contacts and often investing in property of their own.

Nursing has lost that aggressively single-minded, vocational accent, which, virtually by definition, meant that work and family life could not mix. It was a straight choice between career or family, and until quite recently marriage brought an abrupt halt to nursing training or developing a career.

Women may now successfully combine a career and marriage, made possible by a reduction in the working week, improved conditions of employment and the law, easier domestic chores and the whole change in attitude to working women—and married nurses.

The returning nurse may be surprised to see that many more of her colleagues are married women. Their continued employment, prospects of promotion and career enhancement must not be jeopardised by their marital status or motherhood, both of which are protected by the sex equality laws.

Following other trends in society, there are some nurses who are single mothers or divorcees and widows supporting children, while yet others may be caring for aged and ailing relatives at home.

Learners are free to live out, to marry during training and to interrupt their course with maternity leave. At one hospital there is a highly popular and successful course, specifically designed to allow mature students, mostly married women with children at school, to complete general nurse training on a part-time basis. It is interesting to note that this course has a minimal rate of both dropouts and absenteeism, an above-average pass rate in final examinations, and a high proportion of these nurses once they have qualified are retained.

Men in the nursing profession

Anyone returning to nursing would be immediately aware of the notable increase of men in the profession. Although males have traditionally made up a high proportion of the nursing staff in the fields of psychiatry and mental handicap, general nursing was not seen as a job befitting a red-blooded man.

Yet, with nursing having shed its quasi-religious, maid-servant-to-the-doctor image, and assumed the stance of a profession with exciting career prospects, it became an acceptable job for men. Not only acceptable but positively attractive, when there seemed so little competition from female nurses, who had limited career expectations and were likely to be tempted away by marriage and babies.

It is generally assumed that the sex equality laws have bene-fited females in male-dominated professions, yet in nursing the reverse is true. Men, as never before, are clamouring to enter general nursing, making their presence felt in paediatrics and, as a direct result of the Equal Opportunities Act, can now enter for midwifery training at designated schools.

Men have demonstrated ability on a par with their female colleagues to adopt the role of a nurse, bringing with them the brains, brawn, stamina and compassion required. And with their sights set on a career pattern, they head straight for the top positions of power and salary, with little to stand in their way.

Whereas only one in ten students and only one in five registered nurses is male, they currently occupy nearly half of the top jobs in management and education. They are strongly represented as leaders in the health service unions, despite these having a predominantly female membership. Even the RCN, which did not admit men to its membership until 1960, has a large number of men in senior posts, as well as the first-ever male general secretary. Likewise the UKCC, the statutory body representing nurses, has almost as many male senior appointees as female ones.

Indeed, the promotion of men is completely disproportionate to their numbers in the profession. Of course there is no great mystery attached to their meteoric rise up the career ladder. Men, as the breadwinners, are freely able to change jobs, chase opportunities, take on extra responsibilities and studies, supported by wives, who encourage their husbands to charge onwards and upwards—and keep the children out of his way when duty calls, unlike their sister colleagues, who may be hindered by the distraction of marriage and maternity on their career, and are inhibited geographically by their husbands' work.

In many respects the increased male input in nursing has had beneficial spinoffs for the profession. It is suggested that their presence has broadened the outlook of nursing—and nurses— while adding clout to the whole idea of professionalism. In a knock-on effect, these developments have attracted men to the occupation, with which they can now identify and find a suitable niche.

Yet, there is underlying concern of this male over-representation within nursing. The implication is that men, by dominating posts of greatest influence, will create a visible role model. Other men, entering the profession will aspire to aim clearly for the top jobs, demonstrably occupied by males. And the new boys may be given a favourably welcoming hand by those men already up there, in subconscious collusion of that ideal. Females, therefore, especially married ones who have had a substantial break in their career and still have ongoing family responsibilities, will not readily identify with the male-dominated echelons.

The ultimate fear for the future is that females, once again, may be relegated to doing the 'womanly work of caring' at the lowest grades, dominated as before by a male hierarchy.

(It is of course arguable whether this situation represents a male takeover or a female giveaway!)

Cultural and ethnic groups

The nursing population includes a wide variety of cultural and ethnic groups, reflecting those of the general society, and it is good that these patients are represented by like-minded health workers.

At a time when Britain was short of nurses, learners were recruited directly from overseas, leaving a legacy of qualified nurses, mainly originating from Malaysia, Philippines, Maur-itius, Guyana, West Indies and Ireland. General immigration, predominantly from the West Indies and the Indian subcontin-ent, swelled the population of Great Britain, and their children, as British citizens, may choose to become nurses.

In both the nurse and patient populations, there is a wide array of cultural and religious variations, which must be under-stood, respected and catered for. It is mutually beneficial if nurses from the same background can work with patients belonging to ethnic minorities, as they have a special comprehension of the social nuances and perhaps speak the same language. For example a community psychiatric nurse able to speak Gujarati would be of immense benefit in an area with a high Indian population, or a health visitor could be well placed to educate Indian mothers as regards child care and family planning.

Nurses are also bound by their own moral and religious beliefs and may find it unacceptable to work where abortions take place or in a family planning clinic or be involved in blood transfusions. There may be certain religious observances to which she must adhere, such as Jews avoiding non-kosher foods and requesting religious holidays, Muslims observing the fasting at Ramadhan or Sikhs needing to wear trousers or a turban.

Status

In general terms, nurses have a more natural lifestyle, on a par with other employees, who come and go to their job and have plenty of outside interests and varied social contacts. Nurses have a balanced position in society, and nursing is no longer populated by obsessive women with an insular, pathological dedication to duty to the exclusion of all else. The hospital no longer provides the boundaries to a narrow world where elderly spinsters remained cocooned in, and stifled by, the institution, not even knowing the price of a bottle of milk.

Nurses often make early decisions as regards the direction they would like their career to take. Having an established target aim, they choose carefully their subsequent posts and courses of study, in order to pave the way leading either to a clinical specialty, administration, teaching or research.

It is, therefore, not unusual to find senior posts of considerable responsibility occupied by nurses at a relatively young age. The returning nurse may find it surprising, indeed unnerving, to be supervised by a much younger and ambitious colleague.

Conditions in nursing

Since 1981, the full-time employment for nurses constitutes 37½ hours each week. With a need to provide patient care over a 24-hour period, different shift systems are devised to satisfy local requirements.

However, split shifts involving work in the morning and evening with a break in the afternoon are strongly disapproved of, as are 12-hour night shifts. It is appreciated that there are occasions when these may be necessary but they should not be used on a regular basis. Ideally, late evening duties should be restricted to two per person per week and the two days off duty should be allocated together, preceded by an early shift and followed by a late shift, to give the employee a reasonable break. Trained staff usually expect to have alternate weekends off, or one weekend in three.

The concentrated staff ratios during the afternoon period have demanded some reallocation of work schedules away from the traditional morning rush. This period of overlap is also useful for teaching sessions for the staff.

A whole variety of duty rotas are in operation, many needing considerable juggling in order to patch in the odd hours of part-time staff. Ward sisters with a good supply of full-time staff may be able to organise a fixed rota to cover the ward, so that nurses have shifts allocated fairly and know their off-duty days for weeks in advance. Although the lines are fixed, nurses may arrange to do a mutual swap with a colleague.

One example of a duty rota could be as follows:

Day shift

M	T	W	T	F	S	S
Late	Early	DO	DO	Late	Early	Early
Early	Late	Early	Late	Early	DO	DO

where,

Early = 7.45 am–4.30 pm
  (half-hour coffee, three-quarters-hour lunch)   = 7½ hours
Late = 12.30 pm–9.15 pm
  (half-hour tea, three-quarters-hour supper)   = 7½ hours
                    Total 5 × 7½ = 37½ hours

Night shift
  9 pm–8 am
  (half-hour lunch, half-hour tea) = 10 hours × 4   = 40 hours

(As the nurse works 2½ extra hours each week, she earns an extra night off in the fourth week.)

Some hospitals have adopted a system of internal rotation, to give continuity of service to patients, to apportion night duty evenly and to avoid the 'us and them' conflict that sometimes develops between permanent day and night staff. Every nurse is expected to work a spell of day duty, alternating with a period of night duty on her ward, to give continuous cover in rotation.

When the nursing complement is high, with plenty of full time staff and learners, then internal rotation can work well. However, it is not easy to administer with a large number of part-time nurses, and the hospital may lose potential married women keen to return to nursing who would be unable to fit night duty in with family commitments.

The idea of splitting the 24 hours into three equal shifts—for instance 7–3, 3–11 and 11–7—has not proved popular in the United Kingdom.

Accommodation

Many young nurses, at the outset of their career, are still attracted by the idea of being able to leave home, while enjoying the convenience and relative cheapness of living in hospital accommodation. Later on they may choose to live out, although in inner city areas rented accommodation is scarce and the cost can be prohibitive. In any area it can be unsafe to be out late at night alone and transport may present an added problem, if it is inconvenient, unreliable and time-consuming.

Newly built hospitals do incorporate residential blocks, usually giving priority to junior learner nurses and doctors who need to be on call. But there are proposals to sell much of the older off-site NHS accommodation in the future.

Rent is deducted at source from the nurse's salary, but not food; all meals are paid for as they are taken in the system of PAYE—Pay As You Eat.

The 'home sister', who used to be a trained nurse, has been replaced by the lay *'home warden'* to supervise the administration of hospital accommodation. House rules are within moderation for adult occupants, since all have now attained the age of majority at 18, a different situation from the days when student nurses were not 'adults' until the age of 21. Yet, there can be disquieting consequences when security is lax, threatening the safety of people, possessions and property. This difficulty applies to hospital premises in general, because of their relative ease of access and number of people milling around at any one time, some of whom may be unwelcome intruders.

Uniform

The national nurses uniform has been widely adopted by health authorities, as a simple, unfussy work dress in a sturdy easycare polyester/cotton, that will stand up to frequent laundering. Some of the large, well-established hospitals have preferred to retain their traditional, and often distinctive, uniforms, many of which have a multitude of detachable appendages.

The basic slimline national dress has a long front-button opening, a V-neck with self collar and short sleeves. Additional cuffs, collars, belts and linen aprons have been eliminated, since disposable plastic aprons are in general use. A woven raised check design figures on three coloured backgrounds, which denote varying grades of nurse. A beige, biscuit colour is reserved for untrained, auxiliary nurses. Pale blue is for learners, both student and pupil, whose year of training may be signified by stripes on the caps, or epaulettes or coloured belts, depending on local policy. The white version of the dress is for qualified staff, with an additional buckled belt, red or blue for registered nurses and green for enrolled nurses.

Sisters may wear white or the traditional dark blue uniform. In some hospitals they wear small capes, known as tippets, similar to those worn by nurses in the armed services. Senior nursing staff frequently choose to wear mufti (plain non-uniform clothing), especially when they are not directly involved in clinical duties.

Nurses these days are most likely to wear flesh-coloured hosiery, in preference to the customary black stockings of the past. White tights and shoes have gained favour in certain authorities but require scrupulous attention if they are to remain looking clean. There is no doubt that snagged black tights or scruffy white shoes are the worst kind of uniform and may be the most convincing reason of all to select a natural brown as the colour of choice.

Simple paper caps have largely replaced the elaborate frilled, goffered or pleated linen and net versions of earlier years, although senior nurses still select pretty lace caps as a finishing touch to their apparel.

That nurses love their caps, badges and buckled belts is a well-known fact and many are loath to relinquish these emblems of their role.

An enormous fuss erupted when the newly formed UKCC decided against issuing a state badge for nurses who gained a qualification, as the old GNC had done. Hospital badges continue to be provided to nurses who have trained in their establishment, and these are worn with immense pride by those who consider they are hard-earned pieces of metal and worthy of display.

Many nurses, and especially our American colleagues, decry the need for visible insignia to represent a professional person, in particular the cap as a frivolous, archaic and purposeless piece of nonsense, rather more befitting its origins for a Victorian maid than suitable to a modern professional carer. However, any attempts to dispose of caps always meets with vigorous disapproval from all sides of the profession and the public.

It is perhaps somewhat surprising that trouser suits have not been adopted more widely as a suitable uniform for nurses. Physiotherapists wear trouser suits almost universally, as the obvious sensible and comfortable outfit for practical work which involves a lot of lifting and stretching. Although they have gained some popularity for nurses working in areas like theatre, intensive care units, special care baby units, or isolation units, trouser suits are rarely seen on the general wards.

Inevitably the fundamental question crops up every so often, whether nurses should continue to wear any distinctive type of uniform at all, and if they should seek to perpetuate the insignia of status and grade.

Opponents to the uniform argue that it distances professionals from their clients, creates a barrier to easy communication and may invest or imply greater abilities than the owner actually possesses. In other words, does uniform give automatic, perhaps unrepresentative, kudos and is it an unnecessary symbolism for a professional person, whose worth does not rest on characteristic clothing?

Uniform has been discontinued in some areas of psychiatry and mental handicap and in the community, while nurses working with children usually wear cheery aprons with cartoon motifs.

Whenever uniform is discarded, it raises two practical questions. First, should there be any financial allowance in lieu of uniform, to cover for wear, tear and laundering of clothes. Second, how does one maintain suitable standards of dress, considering some of the flamboyant current fashions!

Those in favour of maintaining the tradition of a nursing uniform point out that a familiar outfit enables patients to easily identify with the staff responsible for their care. In a large establishment it is daunting and confusing not to know whom to approach, so strangers may be reassured to see a person whom they recognise as a nurse.

The most down-to-earth argument is the practical role of a uniform, which takes the brunt of all the soiling and smells that accumulate during the daily toil of any nurse.

Hospital personnel are now used to wearing *name badges*, which are an effective communication tool for the many people with whom they come into contact in any day.

Nurses generally give their name followed by their designation thus:

Miss P. Jenkins Ward Sister	or	Mr N. Birch Senior Nurse/Personnel

This tends to be used more than a tag saying | Sister Jenkins |

The title of Ms is increasingly being chosen by women, instead of opting for Miss or Mrs. Professional women who then marry, having become established and well known in their single capacity, often choose to retain their single name, at least for purposes of their career. Some may adopt the American style of joining their husband's name to theirs, as Ms or Mrs P. Jenkins Birch.

As a final word on the subject of uniform, qualified nurses returning to their role after an absence are often happier to resume duty initially dressed as a learner or volunteer, rather than be identifiable as a trained nurse.

Nursing literature

Contemporary nursing literature can be best summed up by saying, 'it is written by nurses, for nurses, about the work of nurses'.

In bygone days it was only doctors who were considered eligible to write on things medical, as those equipped with sufficient knowledge and authority to expound on clinical material. The result was information delivered in the style of the medical model, heavy on pathology, signs, symptoms, diagnosis and treatment, but with only a brief reference to nursing care. Latterly, the task to modify that for nurse readers rested with the sister tutors, as members of the profession possessing advanced education. Everybody else passively read, inwardly digested and regurgitated the 'gospels'.

Nursing itself has developed considerably as a profession in its own right, with a role identity, markedly separated from the doctors. Nurses themselves have discovered their ability, nurtured their writing skills and gained the confidence to write and share their work with interested colleagues. It is no longer left to the academic, erudite few to put their ideas and opinions into print, but is a useful medium available to any nurse who wishes to make a valuable contribution to the development of the profession.

Books

Those early nursing tomes became the standard textbooks, adopted as course books by nurse training schools, and remained largely unchallenged by competitors. It was virtually an area of literary stagnation, as those traditional works were revised and updated, often to appear in their 16th or 20th edition, to be used by generations of nurses. It was not unusual for such books to be handed down from learner to learner, having many years of continued use.

Although nurses do still like to have one or two core books with which they feel comfortable, they are also encouraged to refer to the wide selection of specialist books that are now available. Nurses are not known to be great book buyers, or particularly enthusiastic readers, but today they have access to more books than ever before.

The changed philosophy of nursing practice spearheaded the

need for books with greater relevance to nurses and the job they actually do, based upon the nursing model of care, the problem-solving approach to care and the implications of the increasing body of knowledge gained through research.

Apart from books which cover basic medicine, surgery and practical nursing, there are publications which cater for the full range of nursing specialties that have evolved. Many of these are designed as companions to the clinical courses arranged by the national boards, such as plastic surgery and burns, oncology, intensive care, geriatric care and many more.

A more recent development has been in books specialising in topics derived from the general spectrum of nursing care and dealt with in depth, such as pain relief, counselling, health education, behaviour modification, the nursing process, research or ethics, to name but a few.

Early examples came from the United States, where nurse publications blossomed through the personal need for nurses to advance their own careers by 'getting published'.

Certainly, publishers in the United Kingdom found a huge, untapped market of learners and qualified nurses which, with the right approach, could amount to big business. Many publishing houses have recognised this potential outlet and are developing a nursing section, much as they have done previously with books for doctors, engineers, sixth formers or any identifiable group of readers.

Initially a lot of American books did reach the British market, as the only ones available at the time. Some are useful, others are intensely theoretical and full of jargon as well as being expensive, whereas others were carefully adapted for the United Kingdom and have become very respected nursing books.

It is now recognised that we do not have to look to the United States for books on nursing, when we have our own nurses, familiar with our own system of care, who are perfectly able to produce the necessary material for the profession.

The returning nurse will undoubtedly blow the dust from her old, well-thumbed textbooks when she first contemplates a return to work. It is useful to become reoriented through a book with which you are familiar, but you will soon find that a lot of clinical material, both medical and nursing, is out of date.

It would be a good investment to select a modern book related to your current specialty, once you know where you are to be allocated or have settled into the job. Do not choose hastily. Ask which books the other nurses have found useful, or there may be a textbook on the ward to which you can refer, or look in the training school library and ask for something the tutor might recommend.

If possible, enjoy a day browsing in one of the specialist medical bookshops, like Foyles or Dillons in London or John Wright and Sons in Bristol, which keep a wide range of nursing textbooks. Remember also, it is worth taking a look at the medical section in the public library, where you will find a selection of nursing books, and some interesting ones written for the lay public to provide useful updated background reading.

Journals

The *Nursing Times* holds the market as the popular weekly magazine for nurses, since the *Nursing Mirror* ceased publication in November 1985 after nearly a century of serving the profession. The RCN send a quarterly journal and a weekly newspaper to their members. Other publications such as *Senior Nurse*, *Nurse Education Today*, *Geriatric Nursing* and *Health Visitor*, cater for a more specific readership within the profession, and there is also literature from the societies within the RCN.

A nursing journal today would bear little resemblance to a copy of 10 or 15 years ago. The style, presentation, pace and content are markedly different and reflect the maturity and development of nursing as a profession (see Figure 9.3).

The *Nursing Times* aims to have an evenly spread, balanced content, to appeal to readers across a wide spectrum. Different issues direct their concentration to one field of care, such as maternity or psychiatry, while still including general features to capture the attention of all nurses.

Clinical material is of exceptionally high quality and there is a generous input of articles on research, management and education, from a variety of contributors. News items, information bulletins and critiques keep a finger on the pulse of changes in and around nursing, the politics of the profession and the health service.

Reviews of books and audiovisual aids keep nurses in touch with current publications relevant to their work. A lively letters page invites comments from readers, which it gets in no uncer-

who are qualified nurses, temporarily or permanently having left the nursing profession.

Nurses employed on a part-time basis do have to pay the full membership fee, so as to qualify for the indemnity insurance cover. However, RCN membership fee can be set as a tax-deductible expense.

A new badge, depicting the 'linked hands' logo of the RCN is available to student members, while the traditional badge remains the one issued to qualified nurses (Figure 9.4).

In addition to the above facilities, members receive a weekly newspaper, the *Nursing Standard*, a quarterly magazine, *Lampada* and an annual report and diary, plus a 'Countdown' discount card.

Today, the RCN is the authority that represents the official voice of professional opinion amongst nurses and delivers their views directly to the government and to the public, via the media.

The RCN is an independent trade union and deals exclusively with the interests of nurses as employees. Approaching half a million members, it is the fastest growing trade union in the country.

Other health service trade unions represent the full breadth of health service employees, so that nurses' opinions are represented along with those of other workers. The main unions which do operate in the health service are National Association of Local Government Officers (NALGO), National Union of Public Employees (NUPE), and the one commonly found in psychiatric settings, Confederation of Health Service Employees (COHSE).

Occupational health

Each District Health Authority should have an occupational health department to deal with the ongoing health and welfare of the staff. Often the head of the department is an occupational health physician, aided by *occupational health nurses*, who may be allocated in various locations within the district.

An occupational health sister is involved in health interviews and medical checks on prospective and new employees. With health supervision, she would monitor anyone with a high blood pressure, diabetes, a skin rash or epilepsy and maintain immunisation programmes.

In collaboration with the *health and safety officer*, she is respon-

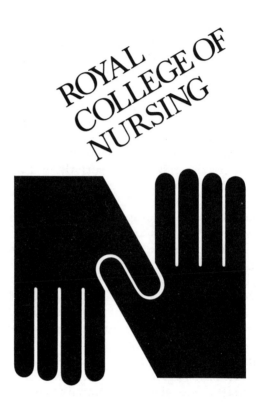

Fig. 9.4   *The linked hands logo of the RCN.*

sible for monitoring environmental factors to ensure a safe place of work for employees. In hospital, this constitutes dangerous practices relating to radiation, fumes, back injury and the disposal of hazardous materials, including foul laundry, clinical waste and sharp objects.

A major component of the role of the occupational health nurse is in health education for all employees, to give advice and instruction on such things as lifting technique, breast examination, relaxation and a good diet. She can also recommend resettlement for staff in a more suitable area of work, such as light duty for someone with a back problem or returning from sick leave.

The occupational health sister also serves an important function as a counsellor. In her autonomous position, she may be the only impartial person whom a nurse can consult about her worries, whether they are of a personal or work-related nature.

As a caring profession, historically, nursing has been notoriously poor about caring and helping when its own members are in any kind of difficulty.

Teaching staff can offer support for learners, newly out of the family nest, unfamiliar with the environment and experiences of caring for people, and finding study difficult. Personnel staff, understanding sisters or nursing officers may also take on the counselling role if approached by a member of staff, yet there may be a problem if the nurse is troubled by some situation at work.

Stress

Stress in nursing is a significant occupational hazard, one that is increasingly being recognised as the cause of much staff absenteeism and repeated minor ailments.

Some areas of care are notably more stressful because of the nature of the work, such as intensive care units, coronary care units, special care baby units, accident and emergency departments, where highly dependent patients are critically ill and nurses are constantly confronted by trauma, pain and death. Stress is equally apparent when a nurse is shouldering weighty responsibility and unsupported, taking on a heavy workload or working long hours for many days consecutively without a break. There may be lack of suitable staff and/or staff dissatisfaction, so she has to cope with the emotional needs of patients, relatives and staff, amounting to intolerable pressure, from which she is unable to escape either physically or mentally.

Nurses working in relative isolation, such as district nurses or health visitors, may experience certain stress, combatting the distressing social and economic circumstances which fuel their workload.

Some authorities, recognising their responsibility to support staff in a positive way, provide a *counselling service*, staffed by trained counsellors, who may also be nurses.

Individual help may be given over personal worries, perhaps with marital or family problems, depression or unwanted pregnancy, and the counsellor can refer her client to a specialist agency if necessary.

Group support is successfully organised to deal with problems arising from work that may be common to many members of staff. It is useful to gather to discuss and air particular grievances, perhaps about pressure of the work environment, learning difficulties, interpersonal relationships or fears for future employment. It is the sharing that provides the caring and the hearing that provides the helping.

A central counselling service, called CHAT, is provided by the RCN for use by any nurse, whether or not she is a member (see page 182).

A new word, recently acquired from the United States, refers to the syndrome known as '*burnout*'. This amounts to a severe form of continued and unalleviated stress, manifest by anxiety, depression, irritability, lack of concentration, leading to a degree of incapacity which prevents the nurse fulfilling her function in a responsible role.

It may occur as a final result of prolonged stress or if a nurse is overburdened with work and study, perhaps being over-zealously ambitious. If adequate support is given when the signs of burnout are first recognised, then it may be prevented, perhaps by suggesting a change of work allocation, a holiday or vocational guidance.

Health problems among nurses

There are two other health problems of considerable concern in the nursing population.

Back injury

The number of working days lost each year through back injury to nurses has been estimated at three-quarters of a million. Some nurses receive permanent damage which renders them incapable of continuing within their chosen profession. Others suffer unnecessary chronic back pain as a result of injury at work.

Employing authorities are required to ensure a safe working environment and to make positive efforts to reduce the incidence of back injury among health service staff. This includes the provision of mechanical handling systems, such as variable height baths and beds, together with demonstration of their correct use. Although these aids may help to alleviate the problem of lifting and transporting heavy, immobile patients, there are many instances where nurses risk back injury by poor manual techniques.

All nurses must have training and supervised practice in patient handling skills and lifting technique, when they join a hospital, either as learners or new staff members, together with periodic instruction thereafter. It is important for them to appreciate how techniques vary for patients in differing circumstances. They must understand how lifting is affected by a restless patient or by one with a certain wound, as well as such dangers as a low bed, an unstable bed or chair, a slippery floor and inequality in the height of the two participant nurses.

A planned programme of training, plus surveillance of environmental hazards and safety procedures, should be reiterated, by employing the services of senior nurses and tutors, physiotherapists and staff of the departments of occupational health, health and safety and health education.

Inadequate staffing levels may cause nurses to take dangerous short cuts and this is a recognised hazard. All things considered, nursing is a high-risk profession for back injuries.

Smoking

As an occupational group, nurses fail badly with a disastrous record as cigarette smokers, apparently unwilling to accept the inherent dangers and showing little inclination to stop. Despite the glaring evidence pointing to the harmful effects of smoking, ranging from heart and peripheral vascular disease, bronchitis and emphysema, cancers of the lung, oesophagus, larynx, mouth and colon, through to stunting fetal growth, nurses show a curious reluctance to relinquish the habit.

By contrast, their medical colleagues have been successful in acting upon their own advice and have ceased smoking in quite dramatic numbers.

Precisely why nurses maintain this recalcitrant stand over cigarette smoking is a matter of interesting conjecture, which invites theories ranging from stress, overwork, boredom, even that they may become blunted to the adverse effects, due to overexposure to sick people.

Whatever the excuses, if nurses are to be worthy and creditable agents of change in the area of health education, they too must heed the warnings and present themselves as models of good health behaviour.

The RCN, in common with many institutions related to health services, has adopted a positive non-smoking policy on its premises.

Retirement

Retirement for the modern nurse should not pose such a devastating alteration in lifestyle, as it did for her institutionalised colleagues of yesteryear. Nevertheless, retirement still presents a notable change after a fulfilling life, spent in a responsible role of caring for others, within the supportive framework of a community environment.

Nurses, like any other employee, may need guidance and advice on how to gain the maximum benefit of their time during retirement. Certainly this period of life requires thought and preparation, with a positive attitude, to achieve the happy, healthy and productive transition from work to retirement.

The Pre-Retirement Association is a general body which provides education, training and advice on this subject. The NHS Retirement Fellowship has a network of active support groups, formed for ex-employees of the NHS of all occupations and all grades.

Many health authorities recognise the need to provide courses in preretirement preparation, particularly since staff can be required to retire compulsorily at the legal age for retirement. This topic is a logical extension of provision of occupational health facilities and may be run by that department or as part of in-service training for staff envisaging retirement.

Reference and refresher reading

Heywood Jones I. (1982). *Sister*. London: W. H. Allen.
Heywood Jones I. (1983). *Senior Sister*. London: W. H. Allen.
  Two novels based upon the true-to-life experiences of a modern nurse working in hospital, to give a picture of what her job really entails.
Kasner K., Tindall D. (1984). *Baillière's Nurses' Dictionary*, 20th edition. Eastbourne: Baillière Tindall.
Middleton D. (1984). *Baillière's Ward Information*. Eastbourne: Baillière Tindall.
Salvage J. (1985). *The Politics of Nursing*. London: Heinemann Medical Books.
Sampson A. C. M. (1982). *The Neglected Ethic: Religious and Cultural Factors in the Care of Patients*. London: McGraw-Hill.

10

Nurse Education

The modern philosophy is of nurse education as a continuous process spanning the whole career of the professional nurse. Education for nurses is no longer confined to the basic period of training and post-basic courses. Although they are of fundamental importance to equip the nurse with basic skills and knowledge, there is plenty more for her to gain in terms of professional development and updating throughout her subsequent working life.

A department of nurse education or a nursing studies unit supervises all the educational programmes within the district, under the director of nurse education (DNE), although programmes may be organised on several hospital sites.

Basic training

At present, courses leading to registration still last for three years, which is now referred to as first level training. From 1986, five 'O' levels will be the minimum entrance requirement for prospective student nurses.

Courses leading to enrolment last for two years and this is known as second level training. To lessen the distinction between students and pupils, the term 'learner' is often preferred to cover both groups, who are obviously in a learning situation and have similar needs for experience.

Certain reductions are available for registered and enrolled nurses who wish to undertake further basic trainings, such as 18 months of psychiatric training, which leads to RMN for the general registered nurse. However, enrolment does not provide a backdoor entry to registration as it once did, by leading fairly automatically to a shortened student training. If enrolled nurses were eligible to become students by virtue of their academic qualifications, a school would undoubtedly expect them to take the full three-year course, however wasteful it may seem.

The ENB does provide a conversion course lasting for one year, to enable enrolled nurses with suitable educational attainments to become registered nurses. Availability of these courses will depend on local need and competition for places is likely to be fierce.

There has been a lot of speculation about the possibility of introducing a single grade of qualified nurse, which might result in the phasing out of the enrolment grade. In anticipation of this idea, some schools have been running down their pupil intakes in favour of increased student groups. Owing to the recession in the jobs market, employers have had no difficulty in filling the larger number of places with suitably qualified student recruits and have concentrated their efforts in this direction.

Until now, prospective nurse learners have had to make application to individual training establishments, which often meant multiple enquiries on their part and duplication of clerical work for schools and those giving references.

From 1986, the ENB hope to set up a *central clearing house* to process all applications for basic trainings, similar to the one which operates for university students.

Individual hospitals would be relieved of the duplication of the initial procedure, but would still conduct interviews and offer places depending on their own criteria of selection. Hopefully this system will give greater efficiency to the selection procedure, reduce clerical work, duplication of forms and medicals, and improve career guidance for the prospective candidate.

It would also reduce the perennial problem of non-attendance by candidates who, having reserved places in several schools, turn up at the one of their choice without bothering to cancel the others, thus leaving gaps in introductory blocks which might easily have been filled.

On the other hand there is tremendous concern over wastage amongst the learner population, with about 30 per cent either failing to complete the course or pass the final examinations.

Even for those who do succeed and qualify there is no guarantee of further employment, which may prove a difficulty for those who are not free to seek work elsewhere. Hospitals are not bound to employ nurses whom they have trained. Their contract ceases once the training course has been completed. During a recession, when staff tend to hold on to jobs, rather than move around, there may be insufficient vacancies to employ the newly qualified nurses, who appear at four or six-monthly intervals in large numbers.

Most training hospitals recognise the difficulty for brand new, inexperienced qualified nurses seeking a job, so they try to honour their commitment to the learners by providing a short-term contract of employment. With three or six months working as a qualified nurse behind her, she is better equipped to seek work on the open market.

Course content

A curriculum is planned around the basic training syllabus, which has been prescribed by the relevant controlling national board. Learners are required to complete a set number of hours tuition, as well as work in certain clinical placements. Learners often know their two or three-year plan of allocations, study blocks and holidays at the outset of their training.

Since joining the EEC, it has been compulsory for all students in general training to have 4 placements: in the community, in geriatrics, maternity nursing and psychiatry, in addition to the general areas of surgery, medicine, paediatrics, theatre or accident and emergency. Considerable clerical work and manpower organisation are involved to provide these allocations, but the trained nurse will be equipped with a wide experience and a balanced view of health care and the services available.

The modular system of training incorporates modules of education, aimed to link nursing theory and practice effectively. For example, in a geriatric module, learners would spend a week in school being introduced to the subject and prepared for their practical placement of six to eight weeks in a geriatric ward or department. Armed with the experience they gained, they return to school for a further week to consolidate their knowledge and skills related to that topic.

All teaching is now based upon the nursing model of care, to enable learners to be involved in total care planning on the wards from the outset of their career. Basic nursing skills are initially taught and practised in the classroom. Wherever possible, these are demonstrated and consolidated in a realistic clinical situation with patients. This is an attempt to bridge the theory–practice gap and hopefully avoid the notorious disparity between what is taught in the school and what is practised on the ward. It is aimed at *patient-centred teaching*.

Clinical instructors (CI), otherwise known as clinical teachers (CT) supervise nurses in a learning situation in their clinical placements and reinforce the theory. This does not interfere with the teaching role of trained nurses, which is built into their job description if they work in an area where learners are allocated.

A recent idea adopted in some institutions is to have someone employed in a joint appointment. She would be a lecturer and a clinical practitioner with a commitment to the service side, in order to retain practical links with the profession and the grass roots aspects of the work.

Throughout the basic syllabus is threaded elements of psychology—the behaviour and experience of individuals, and of sociology—how individuals relate to one another in a social system. There is altogether greater emphasis on the patient as a unique individual, viewed in the context of his social circumstances, on preventive aspects of health care and the role of the nurse in community care.

Basic training includes skills for communication, counselling and teaching, both of patients and colleagues. Nurses are introduced to research appreciation and may even be involved in assisting a research project in a clinical area. Student nurses are given the opportunity to develop their organisational and management skills, through problem-solving exercises and with practice in running the ward, in preparation for when they qualify.

Teaching methods

It has been said that there is no such thing as 'teaching', only 'learning'. A lecturer may speak until she is blue in the face but there is no guarantee that a student has understood or absorbed what she has said. Learning is an active process, which must involve the student. So the true role of an educator is to facilitate the learning process, by directing the student to acquire knowledge and apply it appropriately. Gone are the days of delivering factual lists of information in rote, parrot fashion, without any underlying comprehension.

Of course there will be some requirement for instruction of new skills but much is achieved by self-directed learning, projects, care studies and discussion. The nurse is expected to take greater responsibility for her own education, to work on her own, to make use of books and audiovisual aids, to discuss matters with colleagues, to make her way through worksheets. The tutor acts as a guide and a source for reference, to point the learner in the right direction.

The returning nurse may be surprised to find the modern learner full of confidence, keen to enquire and not shy to ask for explanations, as her predecessors might have been. The learner is encouraged to make best use of the experience throughout her training on her own initiative, rather than being timid and needing to be educationally spoonfed.

Experiential learning

It is always an edifying experience for any health care professional to become patients themselves. Nurses invariably think of themselves as much better in their role once they have been admitted for surgery or had a baby, and realise just how it feels to be on the receiving end.

In a modified way, it is useful for nurses to try to understand the patients' point of view and this can be achieved through experiential learning—perhaps being bathed by colleagues or having to spend a day being nursed in bed, wearing a plaster cast or trying to get around on crutches or a wheelchair, having a nasogastric tube passed or simply balancing on a bedpan. Exposure to these experiences can enhance the nurse's understanding of how the unsuspecting patient might feel and react.

Audiovisual aids

The modern lecturer has a battery of audiovisual aid (AVA) equipment to aid her task of stimulating the interest and motivation of learner nurses. Use is made of the overhead projector to deliver clear writing and diagrams, educational films and tape-slide programmes. Many schools now have a video recording machine, to tape relevant television programmes or to purchase and borrow from the growing stock of video material being designed for the nurse education market. With a video camera, staff are able to record learners in role play, to discuss and evaluate their performance on replay.

Academic gaming

Some inventive teaching can be achieved through academic gaming, a method whereby board games and card games can be used to simulate practical situations and stimulate problem-solving.

Computer-assisted learning

Computers have made their impression on nurse education and, where applicable, learners would need to be introduced to computer literacy to make use of the equipment. Computer-assisted learning (CAL) is an exciting method of teaching and learning by the use of programmed instruction and assessment, which can be adapted to suit individual needs and progress.

Programs are devised by using simulated clinical situations, made plausible by the clout of life-like problems. The nurse must identify the patient's needs and attempt to resolve nursing problems in the safety of the classroom. She is guided through the decision-making process, by a programmed input of knowledge, matched by assessment of her understanding. The nurse is required to contribute throughout, so the machine holds her concentration. If her attention wanders and she fails to respond, her learning experience ceases automatically, unlike the lecturer who carries on regardless!

By recording the progress of the learner throughout the program, the tutor is able to assess and rectify areas of weakness in the learner's knowledge.

Learners often prefer this method to conventional lectures, as they can repeat material when necessary, work at their own pace and at a time convenient to them. Contrary to the passive learning from a lecturer, a learner is actively involved in responding to the computer and benefits by being rewarded instantly with immediate feedback, either boosting her confidence if successful, or stimulating her to try again if she is wrong.

CAL is an aid to education. It does not obviate the use of teachers but relieves them from repetitive lectures, in order to devote their limited time to individual tutorials. Computers do not tire or get bored and they can be amended to keep up to date. They are completely impartial, do not have off days and have infinite patience with learners!

Experience shows that learners like CAL, once they have become proficient in the use of the technology. They take to study readily, enjoy the personalised instruction, the instant feedback and the control they have over their learning. Learners complete their course material more quickly and find they can easily apply their knowledge to clinical practice.

CAL is an effective way of motivating learners by offering a challenge.

Several agencies have set themselves up as resource centres for the audiovisual aids available to augment nurse training. In the future we may even see health education programmes broadcast through the cable television network.

The modern nurse is not being taught to be a task automaton but is being trained to make reasoned judgements and authoritative decisions on patient care. She must be encouraged to use her initiative, think for herself, be enquiring and resourceful and understand the wider implications of health care. Her period of basic training should equip her with the skills and knowledge, to enable her to develop into a professional member of the health care team, responsible for her decisions and actions.

Evaluation of competence

Evaluation techniques must test the knowledge and skills expected that the nurse would acquire, having undergone a period of prescribed training.

Examination for the general register comprises a series of ward-based assessments and a final state essay paper and multiple-choice question paper.

Ward sisters, charge nurses, tutors and clinical teachers undergo an *Art of Examining course*, organised locally, and the DNE will approve successful trained nurses as qualified assessors.

Assessments
In general training, students have four compulsory assessments in which they must be passed competent within their training:

- medicine round
- aseptic technique
- total care of one patient during a span of duty
- management of the ward during one span of duty

Other parts of the register and roll have a modified version of these assessments, to reflect their different syllabus content.

The final examination is currently set and marked by each of the four national boards for training institutions within their country of responsibility. On passing this examination, the nurse is then qualified to apply for registration or enrolment with the UKCC.

Essay papers

A traditional essay paper tests the nurse's ability to evaluate the needs of patient care through from admission to rehabilitation, in view of his lifestyle and social circumstances. Here are two examples of general nursing:

- Arnold Templer, a 70-year-old widower, is admitted for a below-knee amputation of his left leg, due to progressive diabetic gangrene affecting his toes. Discuss the physical nursing care and psychological support this patient will require during the immediate preoperative and post-operative period.

- Four year old Tony is to be admitted to the children's ward for a tonsillectomy. His mother will be resident with him in the cubicle. Discuss how Tony and his mother can be helped to settle into the ward on the day of admission. Discuss how the needs of Tony's mother should be met on the day of surgery.

Multiple-choice questions

Multiple-choice question papers (MCQ), also called objective questions, have gained in popularity because there is no subjectivity related to their marking, as there inevitably will be for essay questions.

The stem poses a question, and there is only one correct answer out of four alternatives. The other three are called distractors, for the obvious reason that they have to be near enough to provide possible alternatives to a sufficient number of students. Devising multiple-choice question papers is not easy and any that are used for examination purposes must be evaluated beforehand by testing on a random selection of likely candidates. Any answer that is obviously too easy is of no use, neither is one that is too difficult—it must be a fair test of knowledge.

Multiple-choice question papers are a useful measure of pure factual knowledge, particularly in areas such as anatomy, physiology and pharmacology. Another benefit is that they can be marked by a computer because there is only one right answer. They are, however, of less value when a definitive answer is not forthcoming, when a variety of factors need to be taken into account or there is a matter of priorities in decision-making. Here follow a few examples of multiple-choice questions. Select *one* answer from (a) to (d).

- Following a total hip replacement, the patient has a drainage tube in the wound. This should be removed,
  (a) in 24 hours
  (b) in 72 hours
  (c) when drainage ceases
  (d) with the sutures
- Which one of the following would be the first aid treatment of bleeding from a deep cut in the forearm?
  (a) apply a tourniquet to the upper arm
  (b) elevate the arm and apply compression bandage to the wound
  (c) catch bleeding vessels with artery forceps
  (d) organise a blood transfusion

(Answers are on page 211).

Continuous assessment

In the future district training schools may be permitted to be responsible for evaluation of their own learners, thus obviating the need for a state final examination. Continuous assessment throughout the course of training is a popular choice, one already employed in some areas of general education.

Throughout each clinical allocation, the learner is supported, guided and supervised by trained members of the nursing staff. Progress reports may form part of continuing assessment, used not for chastening criticism but as a helpful tool to direct the learner to correct and appropriate performance.

Formal planned assessment takes place at suitable intervals for itemised activities, such as removal of sutures, admitting a patient, applying a plaster or organising staff allocation. This gives the learner the opportunity to demonstrate her capabilities and to prove that she has achieved the learning objectives of the training programme.

Assessment of theoretical knowledge and its application to practice is tested throughout the course by means of essays, objective tests, project work and care studies.

There may or may not be a final test on completion of the course. If there is, it should not be the means on which the whole of the nurse's career depends. The aim of continuous assessment is to dispense with terminal, pass or fail type of examination. Ideally, it should ensure that standards of performance are maintained evenly throughout the course, with little variation by peaks and troughs of activity. Any unsuitable candidate could be weeded out along the way, thereby leaving those who complete the course to receive automatic recognition of their sustained achievement.

This also eliminates that absurd situation where a good nurse fails at the final hurdle of the state examination. If she cannot express herself on paper or goes to pieces with examination nerves, she is penalised by failing written work, which immediately invalidates two or three years' excellent work. By the same token, the inconsistent and inadequate nurse, who may be totally unsuited to nursing, could manage to sail through examinations by mugging up on data and technique.

Post-basic training

During the 1960s there was an increasing move towards specialism in various areas of nursing, which demanded a period of training further to basic courses. Individual hospitals set up their own specialist training courses for qualified nurses and awarded a certificate on completion. There developed a random assortment of courses of varying lengths and quality, and their validity was unsure beyond the bounds of the immediate hospital providing training.

Many of the courses did not have well-defined teaching objectives. Some consisted solely of on-the-job experience with a few additional lectures. It is true to say that courses sprang up as a keen way of attracting qualified staff. Clearly there was a need to have some national standard for post-basic training courses, so these became organised under the central body of the Joint Board of Clinical Nursing Studies (JBCNS), formed in 1970.

The JBCNS was among those bodies which were dissolved in 1983, with subsequent supervision of post-basic specialist training handed as the responsibility of the respective national boards. A wide range of clinical courses is now offered to qualified nurses in specialty subjects and skills.

The longer full-time courses, leading to the award of a Certificate, vary in duration from two to 18 months. Nurses generally expect to be employed by the authority which is running the course, but cannot be guaranteed a job once the course has been completed. Alternatively, a nurse may be seconded by her parent hospital, if they feel her position would substantially benefit by the specialty training.

Shorter, part-time courses of study days and/or weeks provide the nurse with a Statement of Attendance or Competence on completion. These are largely organised for nurses who are already employed in a particular area and wish to sharpen their knowledge, be updated on current trends and consolidate their practical experience.

Any training school that wishes to offer a course must comply with the carefully dictated theoretical and clinical objectives, as well as having adequate practical allocation, in order to provide a comprehensive educational programme.

Certificates and statements are awarded by the national boards, although the training school is responsible for the evaluation and assessments of the members' competence and performance throughout the course.

Clinical courses are very popular and competition may be intense for the few places available in any school. Candidates are generally required to have some post-basic experience and preference may be given to those who have shown a particular interest in the specialty and have possibly been working in that type of nursing.

A full list of current courses is included in Appendix 2.

Continuing education/professional development

Basic training for the nurse provides the fundamentals of education, upon which to build throughout her future career. Getting the qualification is not the end of learning, but the beginning, as any trained nurse will verify. Nurses must continue to grow professionally, keep up to date with current trends, and maintain their interest and motivation. Failure to do so will result in stagnation, institutionalised thinking, disinterest and job dissatisfaction.

Continuing education, alternatively called professional development or in-service training, is usually a responsibility allotted to a senior member of staff, to cater for the needs of all staff within a hospital or district authority.

Obviously there are some topics on which every nurse needs to be informed, to ensure she is a safe practitioner, such as laws relating to drugs, lifting technique, disposal of contaminated waste and cardiopulmonary resuscitation.

In-house courses or study days may be arranged on subjects of general interest in nursing and health care, making use of district personnel as speakers to share their expert knowledge. Items would include those mentioned in the plan for a refresher course (see Figure 4.2), as a way of stimulating interest in working nurses: stoma care, pain control, bereavement, community provisions, joint disease, cancer treatment, the list is endless. Yet some ongoing education is necessary for nurses who perhaps, by virtue of their domestic circumstances, are not in a position to chase regular career opportunities or seek higher positions.

Special needs may need to be served for nurses who may be involved in interviewing, counselling or need to attend an Art of Examining course in order to assess learners. Nurses working in specialist areas may need training in certain skills, such as intravenous drug additives, use of a defibrillator or reading an ECG.

Staff could enhance their knowledge by visiting related institutions, perhaps a day centre for the elderly, an adult training centre for the mentally handicapped, or the Disabled Living Foundation, which has a wealth of items and information to assist the physically disabled.

Nurses could swap allocations to gain alternative clinical experience or be assigned to work alongside a trained nurse in a different field of care, such as accompanying a district nurse or health visitor for a few days, to give some greater insight into their role.

Many schools now make use of video material and Open University packages, as a way of widening the learning opportunities for their qualified staff.

There are plenty of outside conferences and courses of interest to nurses, arranged by organisations, goods manufacturers, hospitals and professional journals. These are widely publicised and nurses are obviously eligible to attend independently. Or they may hope to get financial assistance and study leave, although this is dependent on the policy of their employing authority, rationing of resources and sympathetic understanding of the professional needs of their staff. The same constraints apply to secondment for post-basic clinical courses and assistance for diploma and degree courses.

Staff appraisal

Staff appraisal enables senior managers to discuss a nurse's progress and performance at work, to highlight good and not such good areas which could be improved upon. It is also a good time to talk about career prospects and the opportunities for the nurse in the way of continuing education.

At present, continuing education is a rather hit-and-miss affair. You may be lucky to work for a progressive, enlightened and generous authority—or you may not. Part-time nurses and those with a nurse bank or agency may be at a disadvantage for being included in educational ventures, even though their needs are of equal importance as their full-time contemporaries.

The situation is set to change in the future, when the UKCC link evidence of updating as a prerequisite for periodic relicensing (see page 87). Hopefully, this will result in greater provision of educational opportunities for nurses, although the onus may rest on the staff to take responsibility for their own professional development, which involves commitment of their own time and money.

Diploma in Nursing

Since 1926, the Diploma in Nursing (DipN) has provided a course leading to an advanced qualification in the knowledge and skills of nursing practice. There was a steady, although modest, throughput of students annually until the 1960s and 1970s, when the demand suddenly increased. Attention to the DipN coincided with the greater emphasis on higher academic qualifications, resulting in an enormous and continuing growth of nurses offering themselves for the course of study and examination.

To keep abreast of the radical changes within nursing practice and education, the DipN was subject to a major review, culminating in a revised syllabus in 1981.

The new course comprises six units of learning, normally extending over a period of three years of part-time study. Each unit is tested by course work or written examination before progressing to subsequent units.

Units 1 to 4 provide a broad-based education for the student to widen her knowledge and understanding of nursing. Units 5 and 6 require the nurse to focus her experience on her chosen field of study, to demonstrate a deepened awareness of one particular nursing specialty. An outline of the course content is shown in Figure 10.1.

The curriculum and assessments are controlled and monitored by the extramural department of the University of London, but courses are offered locally and validated by the University.

Programmes are arranged jointly between a college of higher or further education and a school of nursing. There are currently 32 centres approved by the University of London. Separate, though similar, arrangements occur in Wales. Any interested nurse could write to the University for a list of approved centres, then apply directly to the centre of choice to be considered for a place. It would also be worth discussing proposals with the clinical manager, to find out the likely situation with regard to financial assistance and study leave.

Courses are generally organised on a weekly day-release basis. Members will need to be committed to the course, as they are required to do a substantial amount of individual study and to prepare work for assessment. As the course proceeds through the units within the three-year period, student learning becomes increasingly self-directed.

Members joining the course come from a wide variety of backgrounds in nursing and bring different experiences, so there is emphasis on seminars and group work to pool ideas, for the benefit of all.

Candidates for the DipN must be first-level nurses (registered nurses). Course centres are responsible for selecting suitable members, whom they think could manage the study, are likely to succeed in assessments and will profit in their professional development from the course.

They are looking for evidence of clinical competence and an appropriate academic background. As a guideline, they recommend five 'O' levels, but this need not automatically exclude candidates who do not possess the paper qualifications. Alternative admission procedure may comprise an interview and a piece of written work on a professional topic, in order to demonstrate academic potential to pursue the course.

Beyond unit 2, nurses do need to be in some form of employment, even in a part-time capacity, as they are required to complete work based upon clinical application. Fees for the course can amount to more than £100 each year and, although some

1ST YEAR

COURSE UNIT 1

The Human Organism

The characteristics of living
   things
Human development
Differences between
   individuals
The individual and the group
The integrated functioning of
   the human organism
The behaviour of the
   individual

COURSE UNIT 2

Social Organisation and Social Change

Organisation
Concept and nature of society
Social order
Patterns of social change

2ND YEAR

COURSE UNIT 3

The Application of Care

Decision making
Concepts of nursing
Relating care to needs of the
   individual
Comparative systems of care

COURSE UNIT 4

Emergence of Modern Nursing and Midwifery

The nursing role
The responsibility of the nurse
Preparation of the nurse
The nurse as a professional
   worker
Sociocultural influences on the
   role of the nurse
Comparative systems of
   nursing education

3RD YEAR

COURSE UNIT 5

Research and Nursing

The place of nursing research
Research questions and
   problems
Ethical considerations
Statistics
Research methods

COURSE UNIT 6

Nursing

The search for excellence in
   nursing
(a) special age groups
(b) special environments
(c) special forms of nursing
     practice

Fig. 10.1 *Summary of course units of the new Diploma in Nursing. (Reproduced by kind permission of the Extramural Department of the University of London.)*

nurses do fund themselves, most would hope to be seconded by their employing authority.

The DipN provides an accredited foundation for nurses who wish to proceed to further studies and paves the way for degree courses and teaching. Yet the prime objective of the DipN is to enable the nurse to develop as a clinical practitioner within her chosen specialty.

Degree courses

The nurse holding a degree is becoming an increasingly common phenomenon within the profession. Traditionally there has been some scepticism towards highly intellectual people doing what has always been seen as an essentially practical occupation. Sometimes the obstructive thinking developed into feelings of frank animosity, which did nothing to endear bright people to nursing.

Yet with the new wave of professionalism and the firm theoretical basis founded for practice, nursing requires colleagues trained for independent inquiry and in possession of good academic skills.

Nurses with a degree tend to be high achievers through self-motivation. Many do accelerate into teaching and administration, although plenty choose to remain at the grass roots, to excel in clinical practice.

It is a natural extension for the nurse graduate to continue on into research, which is an area badly in need of development within the profession, and the individual nurse will also benefit by gaining a master's degree or doctorate (MSc or PhD).

Another field in which the graduate usually excels is with the skills of communication, both verbal and written, so that their contributions are welcomed at conferences and in nursing literature, to the advantage of all members of the profession.

Despite a slow acceptance of nursing as a discipline, there are now several professors in chairs of nursing as a special faculty within British universities.

A nurse may be involved on a degree course either before, during or after her basic nurse training.

The graduate who chooses to take nurse training subsequent to obtaining her degree may be eligible for a shortened nurse training course at selected centres. She may, however, find the transition from university student to nursing student rather a shock to her system. Having been used to a *laissez faire*, freewheeling style, which relies heavily on individual responsibility to succeed, she will be amazed at the compulsory classroom attendance and periods of practical allocation, which are dictated by the statutory bodies for training.

Also, study must be undertaken alongside physically tiring work and a responsible role on the job. The traditional institution of nursing and its hierarchy is totally at odds with the life on a university campus!

Nevertheless, these are popular courses and many graduates stay the nurse training course and continue in careers within the profession.

Several arrangements for degree courses linked to nurse training have been developed in recent years. As there is only a smattering of such establishments, there is keen competition for the limited places and entrants are required to possess two or three 'A' levels in relevant subjects.

Students pursue a tough theoretical course at the university or polytechnic, interspersed with practical experience based with their parent hospital, frequently occurring during the vacations. Despite a concentrated and demanding course, there are significantly fewer dropouts than from normal nurse training courses.

Following a four-year course, the successful candidate gains a nursing qualification and a degree. Most qualify as RGN but there are a few courses leading to RMN and BSc (social sciences). The degree obtained may be in the specialty of nursing, as Bachelor of Nursing, BSc in Nursing Studies or BSc in Nursing Sciences or a degree of a related topic, such as life sciences, economics, social sciences or social administration.

It has become increasingly popular for registered nurses to study for a degree after gaining their nursing qualification. Senior nurses and tutors, in particular, have demonstrated their desire and ability to undertake degree courses as a form of professional advancement, to enhance their expertise and career opportunities.

Some degree courses are specifically tailored to cater for nurses as undergraduate students, either in pure nursing subjects or in allied disciplines, so that registration becomes one of the prerequisites for applicants. Nurses are also able, as any other citizen, to go to university at a later stage in their life. If they study full-time, they may be eligible for a local education authority grant.

However, senior nurses, with an established position in their profession, may be reluctant to give up work, and their salary, so may prefer to study for a degree on a part-time basis, probably day release over a period of four years. Occasionally, the final year can be taken on a full-time basis, with secondment from the employing authority.

Having obtained a first degree, it is possible to proceed to gain a master's degree or PhD, both of which involve commitment to advanced study and original writing or research.

Open University courses

The Open University has proved a most desirable option for working nurses who wish to study for a degree but remain actively involved with the profession, and for those deciding to grasp the opportunity later in life.

It is flexible and adaptable, requires little in the way of travelling, can be done at home at a pace dictated by the student. However, the work is demanding and it is reckoned to require at least 16 hours of committed study each week to keep up with the course, as well as attendance at summer school. There is continuous assessment throughout the course, which, together with a pass in the final examination gains the student a credit.

A degree is built up by an accumulation of passes known as 'full credits', six for an ordinary degree and eight for an honours degree. Candidates need show no evidence of previous academic attainments and students are accepted largely on a first-come, first served basis, with a slight shuffling to ensure a good balance from the population. Anyone with an advanced nursing qualification, such as Diploma in Nursing or Registered Nurse Tutor, is eligible for an award, which will exempt her from one or part of the credits.

The flexibility is probably its most attractive feature, especially to nurses holding down a demanding job, or for mothers at home with variable commitments. Students may spread the course over any number of years or take a break from study between credits and return at a more convenient time.

This popular system provides study through *distance teaching*, a style based on the idea of a correspondence course. Teaching material is mailed to the student and is augmented by radio and television programmes and tutorials at study centres.

As well as providing degree courses by this method, the Open University have designed a selection of study packs on health and social welfare topics. These are of immense value to nurses in both basic and continuing education, although they are not rewarded by any certificate or credit. They may be purchased by individuals, but are more commonly held by schools of nursing for repeated use in study groups. Study packs include all the necessary teaching material, such as a study guide, individual workbooks, videocassette, resource guide and notes for a group leader. Here are some of the topics currently available which might be of interest to nurses: a systematic approach to nursing care (nursing process); caring for older people; abuse in families; rehabilitation; topics in drug therapy; the handicapped person in the community.

Distance learning is likely to become a feature of nurse education in the future; in 1986 two centres—one in Manchester, the other in London—will begin offering distance learning packages to nurses (see Appendix 1 for addresses).

Nurse teachers

There are two grades of nurse teachers, the registered nurse tutor (RNT) and the registered clinical nurse teacher (RCNT), equal to a registered clinical instructor (RCI) in Scotland.

Any prospective nurse teacher must show evidence of suitable clinical practice before being accepted on any teaching course. This must be two years post-basic experience (exclusive of post-basic training courses) with not less than one year spent in a position of responsibility in a clinical area where learners are regularly trained.

There are two routes of entry for a clinical teacher. A six-month full-time course at any one of a number of centres, leading to the Clinical Teaching Certificate of the Royal College of Nursing. Or, in addition to holding the Diploma in Nursing, a nurse may take the Further Education Teachers Certificate of the City and Guilds of London Institute (FETC, course 730) on a part-time basis.

A nurse tutor candidate will initially need to hold the Diploma in Nursing or a similar advanced professional qualification, together with five 'O' levels. This is followed by secondment to a college for a one-year full-time teaching course, to gain a teachers training certificate, a Diploma in Education or Certificate in Education. This combination equips her with the necessary advanced knowledge of nursing practice, together with teaching method and skills.

Individual colleges which run these courses stipulate their own entry requirements, so they do vary, but most will make alternative arrangements for mature applicants without paper qualifications, who may be admitted at the discretion of the selection panel.

Graduate nurses are often attracted to teaching and are welcomed on these courses because they have a great deal to offer the profession in this sphere.

Having obtained an accredited teaching certificate, the clinical teacher or tutor needs to apply to the UKCC to be registered in these respective positions.

Traditionally, the clinical teacher has largely been concerned with the practical aspects of training, by demonstrating skills, helping learners in their clinical placements and arranging completion of ward-based assessments; whereas the tutor is responsible for the theoretical content of the curriculum and overall planning and organisation of courses.

Originally these two were distinct and separate roles but they have increasingly overlapped, especially with tutors taking a greater part in clinical involvement. The two roles may eventually merge to produce one nurse teacher, causing the ultimate demise of the clinical teacher.

The future of nurse education

Nurse education stands at the crossroads, poised for change to equip the profession efficiently for the future needs of health care. The UKCC is currently engaged upon a total reappraisal of the education and training of nurses in 'Project 2000'. Although it would be presumptuous to attempt any prediction of the outcome, it is likely to result in significant alterations in the current system. Some hot issues are repeatedly being brought into the limelight for discussion.

One persistent call, initially suggested in the Briggs Report, is for one single grade of qualified nurse, with a common core of basic training that lays the foundation for further specialism. There is certainly a need to rationalise some of the wasteful overlap of education occurring when nurses embark on successive training courses.

Enrolled nurses have been particularly concerned about the erosion of their role, both currently and in the future. There is general dissatisfaction with the limited post-enrolment opportunities, both in professional development and with their restricted level of employment. Although she cannot function independently without supervision from a registered nurse, the enrolled nurse is a well-trained member of the team with good experience. Those who possess the qualification can be assured that their position will be safeguarded by incorporating them into any future reorganisation.

It is a contentious matter whether nurse education should concentrate blindly on high academic attainment as the main criterion for student nursing, which would effectively bar those people who have other useful attributes necessary to make a good nurse. Probably there is room in the profession for various contributors.

Another ongoing dispute is whether the nurse learner should be engaged purely in a student capacity, supernumary to staff requirements, so that her presence in clinical areas is devoted to her educational needs. Traditionally, education of the nurse has been inextricably linked with the service side. The apprentice-style system of training involves considerable commitment as an employee contributing to the nursing labour force. It is argued that these demands take a priority and thereby compromise her needs as a learner. If she were a student, remuneration would have to be paid as a bursary or grant, instead of the current training allowance which she now gets as reward for service as a member of the NHS manpower workforce.

If students are disengaged from the nursing service, there may be a need to make a concerted effort to encourage back and retrain those resting qualified nurses. These would be needed to maintain the service, unless the profession is prepared to rely on ever-increasing numbers of untrained personnel giving care at the bedside. Continuing education and professional development programmes are likely to be a key topic as regards retaining and motivating the staff already in employment.

Nurse education may develop close collaboration between

higher and further education outside the hospital environment. Nurse educationalists may eventually be of only one grade, probably in the long term aiming towards graduate nurse teachers, able to work in both the clinical setting and the classroom.

Nursing of the future is bound to reflect the orientation towards health education and preventive care and away from disease. Any proposed changes would need to represent the increasing emphasis on nurses working in the community and generally in developing their role as autonomous practitioners in several areas of care.

Some authoritative documents from various areas in the profession have already put forward suggestions about the future of nurse education. As yet, nothing has been decided but it is certain that the profession faces a crucial and challenging time ahead, no doubt with some radical changes on the horizon.

Whatever system is finally adopted, it is imperative that the UKCC get it correct at the first attempt, because there are unlikely to be any second chances. Before making any definitive decisions, it will make wide consultation within the profession. Nurses will be kept in touch with all proposals and any changes along the way, through the nursing journals and conferences. We can expect to see plenty of lively and heated debate before the dust settles on the future shaping of plans for nurse education.

The UKCC are committed to doing their best for the profession and the public, as they lead nursing into the 21st century.

Answers to multiple-choice questions on page 198 are (c) and (b) respectively.

11
Modern Trends in Health Care

Wherever a nurse is employed, she never works in isolation. She will come into contact with other members of staff, with patients and relatives, who may require help from other health or social services.

The intention of this chapter is to give an overview of the major areas of health care. It shows how changes in ideas and attitudes, together with social, medical and legal developments, have contributed to their present status. Within each field is demonstrated how the nursing profession has adapted to keep in line with modern concepts, reflected in current training programmes and career opportunities.

These sections below attempt to give a flavour of modern trends in health care, to enable the interested returning nurse to update her knowledge on a variety of important topics. None is aimed at definitive coverage of any field of care, and those wishing to look deeper into any specialty are recommended to further reading.

Acute care

Probably *the* most striking feature of acute care that the returning nurse will notice, is the speed with which inpatients are treated and despatched home. Those having major surgery, with a routine, uncomplicated recovery, are likely to be discharged as soon as their sutures have been removed.

The average stay for open-heart surgery for a routine coronary artery bypass graft (the *CABBAGE* operation) is ten days. 'Routine' in this case involves splitting the sternum, being attached to a heart-lung machine, dealing with foreign blood, stopping the pumping mechanism of the heart during intricate surgery, then shocking it to restart, plus a vast laceration from ankle to groin from where a suitable vein is utilised!

Following minor operations, patients may go home even earlier, their stitches being taken out on a return visit or by the district nurse. With such speedy dealings, the patient has limited time for preoperative orientation to the hospital environment, while any convalescent period weighs heavily on the family and community services. Indeed, the whole idea of convalescence is used less and less, having assumed old-fashioned connotations linked with memories of tuberculosis, rheumatic fever, scarlet fever and a darkened room, Benger's food and bone broth.

This is a pity if it trivialises the recovery period following operation or illness. As the thinking goes, once you have been discharged from hospital, the authorities must have deemed you fit to leave and expect you to make rapid progress. Yet, it does a disservice to the patient to underestimate the physical and emotional trauma surrounding a general anaesthetic and surgical assault.

The postoperative patient requires a period of rest and readjustment back to normal health. Those who do make a seemingly speedy recovery may sink into a lethargy and depression some months later, resembling delayed shock or a bereavement reaction. This is not uncommon particularly following major gynaecological surgery.

Early discharge has in its favour that if patients can recuperate gently at their own speed, many would prefer to be in their own home, away from the hubbub of a noisy, busy hospital routine, notorious for disturbing patients' valuable sleep.

Much of the idea behind encouraging rapid progress is based on the sound benefits to be derived from early ambulation. It is now acknowledged that bed is a dangerous place to be, so that getting up and about reduces the incidence of deep vein thrombosis, pulmonary embolism, pressure sores, chest infection, and joint stiffness among other complaints. Virtually all general surgical patients sit out of bed on the day following operation. There have also been dramatic changes in the gentle early mobilising of patients after eye surgery and following a coronary thrombosis, both of which traditionally spent long periods in bed, with limited activity.

Early ambulation is all the more important because there is a higher proportion of elderly patients needing acute care, who must be firmly moved towards rehabilitation if they are not to become irrevocably immobilised. The high incidence of older people in the population of any general medical or surgical ward will be another conspicuous feature of modern hospital life to the returning nurse.

As far as the staff are concerned, a rapid turnover of patients generates a considerable increase in administrative work, in admission and discharge procedures, taking a nursing history, medical clerking and the routine list of tests and investigations. There is extra work for clearing and making new beds, as well as exceedingly heavy operation days, with a lot of high-dependency patients at any one time.

The major implication is that nurses may fail to get work satisfaction from care delivered in treadmill fashion, when they are unable to develop ongoing nurse/patient relationships. Both the nurse and the patient may suffer when a hospital experience is reduced to the impersonal delivery of routine care.

The returning nurse will also recognise a change in emphasis on disorders, diseases and treatments. There is less concern about the old-style infective and infectious conditions or their sequelae, like rheumatic fever and heart disease, measles and meningitis or kidney failure from streptococcal infection. Even tuberculosis, when it makes an occasional appearance, is quickly arrested by drug therapy, which continues on an outpatient basis.

Surgery pioneered 20 years ago has become routine today, because we have the technology and the safety of support systems, such as transplants of bone marrow, cornea or kidney, plastic surgery operations and all manner of surgery to the heart, by courtesy of the extracorporeal circulation.

Recovery area

Most hospitals have a recovery area attached to the theatre suite, where all patients are supervised until they have regained consciousness and their observations are stable. It is no longer advisable to allow patients to return to their ward in the unconscious state, for fear of crisis occurring en route.

Postoperative patients are placed on a trolley and wheeled to the responsible recovery ward nurse, who has emergency equipment at hand, including piped oxygen and suction machinery. The anaesthetist is also nearby and will check each patient before permitting them back to their general ward.

Anaesthetic nurses

Also appointed to work in recovery and the anaesthetic room is the anaesthetic nurse, a relatively new role which is served by a clinical course. She is designated to the management and care of the patient being prepared for, undergoing and recovering from anaesthesia and may go to visit him in the preoperative phase. She works alongside the anaesthetist and her duty may extend to be included on the cardiac arrest team, which is called out for resuscitation anywhere in the hospital.

Recovery is a busy area, with a continuous throughput of dependent patients requiring careful supervision, following any one of a variety of surgical procedures. The job is confined to fairly regular daytime hours and offers scope for part-time employment, which may be attractive to the returning nurse with home commitments.

Day surgery

Yet another interesting move is towards more day surgery. It is increasingly popular as a way of reducing the long waiting lists for elective surgery and has been made possible because of superior modern anaesthetics, whose effects wear off much more quickly than earlier preparations.

Day surgery may be organised so that patients are added to the theatre list and nursed during the day in an ordinary surgical ward. Or there may be a special day surgery unit, with its own theatre and own staff committed to the preoperative and postoperative care on a daily basis. Staff work either an early or late shift to cover both ends of the day but there is no night allocation, which makes day surgery very cost-effective. Should a patient not be fit for discharge by the evening, as rarely happens, he would be admitted to a general ward overnight.

Day surgery would be suitable for conditions such as excision of lipoma, carpal tunnel decompression or dental extraction, as well as small operations on children. There is also an increase in investigative procedures carried out on an outpatient basis, so nurses may be employed in endoscopy units, scanner units or to help with barium studies in X-ray, or amniocentesis or ultrasound examination.

Five-day ward

Midway between day care and an ordinary stay is the concept of the five-day ward, providing 24-hour staff cover from Monday morning through to Friday evening, but closed at weekends. This is an appropriate arrangement for patients having longer tests or small operations, like minor gynaecological or rectal surgery, when they require only a few days in hospital or have no one at home to care for them.

Intensive care

Intensive care nursing has been a major growth area in acute care since the 1960s, when machines paved the way to control lifegiving respiration. Subsequent developments with mechanical ventilation and intravenous feeding techniques have resulted in the utopian ideal of the 'life-support system'.

Patients requiring intensive care need highly skilled nurses to perform the many procedures and observations relating to this specialty. As the key member of the team, by providing constant surveillance of patients' conditions, she carries a tremendous weight of responsibility for the outcome of care in the intensive care unit. Certainly, intensive care regimens have succeeded in giving spectacular results with critically ill patients, as well as making possible advanced surgical techniques that would previously have been unthinkable.

A unit with specialist equipment and trained staff may be called an intensive therapy unit (ITU) or intensive care unit (ICU). The American term of 'critical care nursing' is beginning to creep into British usage and is a familiar term found in books from the United States. It is recommended that a district general hospital should have one intensive care unit bed for every 100 of its general bed complement, to serve those patients who are critically ill. They may be transferred from any ward or department, from accident and emergency, or directly from theatre, dealing with a wide range of grave conditions including trauma, cerebral catastrophe, drug overdose, aortic aneurysm or postsurgical emergencies.

Beds may be allocated for patients with medical heart problems, mainly myocardial infarction, or be in a separate coronary care unit (CCU). Hospitals which concentrate on any specialist types of surgery will have an accompanying specialist intensive care unit, such as postcardiac surgery, postrenal or hepatic surgery or neurosurgery. Other specialist units will nurse patients in a reverse barrier situation, when they need to be protected from infection and to remain in a sterile environment, as, for instance, burns victims or those having immunosuppressive drugs.

Because there is always pressure on the limited number of beds in intensive care units, it is only the most dangerously ill patients who warrant entry. They are invariably totally dependent, supported by all manner of drips, drains, pipes and probes, every aspect of their condition requiring close monitoring. Nurses are trained to be conversant with the associated high-tech equipment they commonly use: resuscitation procedures, tracheostomy and ventilator care, interpretation of ECG tracings, handling of multiple intravenous infusions, central venous pressure and arterial lines, in addition to basic care of the patient. Their work frequently encompasses the extended roles of the nurse, such as giving intravenous additives and defibrillation.

There is, however, a definite danger that the interpersonal needs of the patient may become neglected if the technical work assumes greater importance and the nurse becomes engrossed and overwhelmed by her many systematised duties with machines and monitors. Great emphasis has been placed on the necessity to communicate with and reassure patients, many of whom may be unable to respond because they are intubated or unconscious, but may be perfectly able to hear. They still require the human warmth and contact, probably even more than other patients, because they are in alien surroundings, have lost control of their bodily functions and been overtaken by the impedimenta of the intensive care unit, as well as being in mortal fear for their future wellbeing.

A stay in the intensive care unit is extremely stressful for patients. For despite the obvious benefits to their physical health, many find the claustrophobic experience intolerable, complaining then and later of nightmares, hallucinations, disorientation, anxiety and depression. During their stay they are subjected to sensory deprivation from loss of tangible indicators of time and place; the lights are always on, there is no distinct day or night, no mealtimes to shape the day. They also suffer from sleep deprivation from disturbances in the environment, routine continuous observations, a trail of doctors, physiotherapists, X-ray technicians and strange noises from the machines.

In fact it has been shown in several surveys that heart attack patients nursed and supervised at home are likely to have an equally good prognosis as those nursed in a high-tech unit, where the trauma of admission can increase anxiety.

Working in the intensive care situation can be stressful for nurses too. Some hospitals recognise this by giving their intensive care unit nurses a spell away from the unit, to work for a while in a general ward.

The very nature of intensive care nursing involves being in a highly emotionally charged situation on a continuous basis. *Every* patient is seriously ill, with the potential to get much worse. The nurse encounters a high level of morbidity and a higher-than-average mortality rate, and it can be distressing and demoralising to witness a string of deaths. Nurses miss the joy of seeing a patient through to discharge for, as soon as any patient makes suitable progress, he is transferred to a general ward, to make way for the next critically ill patient.

There is no lull when nurses can chat to a resting convalescent patient. As intensive care unit nurses are incessantly confronted by patients in the gravest of circumstances, it is vital that a unit has good team work, with supportive staff relationships conducive to maintaining a high staff morale. The intensive care unit nurse carries the responsibility that her instantaneous response and action can be crucial to the outcome of a life or death situation.

Learner nurses may be allocated to gain experience in intensive care units, but only in a supernumary capacity, always working alongside a trained unit nurse. It is an experience guaranteed to provide a new perspective in care, one that will contribute to the learner's confidence and maturity, albeit daunting at the outset.

Intensive care nursing is a highly specialised area of care, served by a post-basic clinical course of training. It is an interesting area and provides plenty of challenges, but would not be the obvious place for the returning nurse, until she has been suitably updated and is given on-the-job instruction and supervision.

Continuing care

The use of the words 'chronic', 'terminal' or 'long stay' when applied to care, reflect a dismissive, hopeless attitude to the patient's outlook. By portraying a fatalistic approach, these words may imply that the person is less deserving of comprehensive attention, and is at a stage where he can only expect to receive second-class care.

So the concept of 'continuing care' tries to instil a more positive, encouraging ring to the ongoing needs of those with a chronic illness or disability, terminal disease or the elderly infirm. Because, even though curative medical treatment has ceased, each patient can benefit from supportive nursing care, preventive measures and rehabilitation, to help them live the remainder of their lives in contentment.

Continuing care is effected in units designed either for the young disabled, or those with severe mental handicap, or for the elderly infirm in a variety of settings, as well as in the community for everybody in need. Personalised care is geared to meet the special needs of that individual, to help him achieve the maximum of functional ability and social integration, and also his potential for self-care.

The person who is dying in a busy hospital frequently receives somewhat superficial attention, amidst the flurry of general activity and the urgent needs of acutely ill patients. Indeed, in an environment where the accent is on recovery and good health, death may be seen as a failure of the curing service, and the dying person equally dismissed as a failed case. We have all seen the terminally ill patient being moved gradually up the ward, then into the side room, out of sight, left to fade away in isolation, dying in solitude.

Hospice movement

The hospice movement is dedicated to caring for the dying person and his family. Their pioneering work has impressed on all health workers the need for positive ideals which enable the dying person to spend his final days in a loving, tranquil, untroubled existence. Family members too are encouraged to stay with their relative and are helped to overcome their own fears and distress surrounding the parting at death.

Crucial to the care of the dying is the need to control the harrowing symptoms that often accompany terminal illness, such as pain and vomiting. It is this suffering that people fear, more than the act of dying itself. The aim is to offer pain relief without drugging the person into an uncontrolled, mindless oblivion or hastening an untimely death. Pain control goes side by side with the physical, emotional and spiritual support. In a hospice, no person is ever left to die alone or shunted out of view, someone is always there at that final moment of darkness.

Where the dying person can be cared for at home, the 'hospice at home' service extends their expertise to help relatives and the community services, by providing emotional support and practical help, often in the form of a visiting nurse. By sharing the experience with understanding professionals, the relatives may be helped to cope in what is, undeniably, a most agonising situation.

There is at least one hospice dedicated to the care of dying children and their families. It is the aim of all hospices to give some continued support and comfort to relatives in their time of bereavement after the patient has died. It is a natural extension of their role, having developed an intimate and sensitive relationship over the previous months.

Far from being a gloomy, sad or despondent place, a hospice is filled with an aura of love and serenity, dedicated to the satisfying task of ensuring a peaceful, pain-free death, which ordinary hospitals often find difficulty in providing.

As the dying man said, 'Dying may be a routine business for you, nurse, but it is the first time for me'.

The returning nurse may find continuing care a gratifying place to work, where there is emphasis on basic skills and the development of ongoing relationships, well suited to a woman with the fortitude and mature outlook derived from life experiences.

Care of the elderly

During the heady days of medical expansion in technology, with new drugs, treatment regimens and surgical advances, 'cure' assumed the paramount importance in health care. The mundane, unspectacular care of the elderly fell from public and professional gaze, except for rashes of publicity about ill-treatment. But on the whole, how could the day-to-day routine of an incontinent, demented old man or woman hope to capture headlines monopolised by the glory of life-prolonging transplants and cancer therapy, which drew victims back from the jaws of death?

The status of the geriatric patient was at an all-time low,

equalled only by the status of the geriatric nurse, considered to be working in an uninspiring, uneventful, unimportant area of care. Where no great advances could be expected, no sensational challenges to be overcome, geriatric nursing as a specialty had little to offer in the way of career advancement. It was, literally, at the bottom of the professional heap, often seen as a job to be relegated to untrained staff, or to nurses who were supposedly content to 'tick over' rather than exert themselves in a demanding field of employment.

The negative attitude to the elderly effectively dismissed them as an unworthy cause, somewhat low on the priority of the *serious* business of health care. Implicit in this idea was that those near the end of their life did not deserve as much effort or expenditure as younger people with plenty of life left. It was an attitude that filtered through society as well, embodied in the glorification of youth.

Now, with the 'quality' of life taking an equal stance alongside the 'quantity' of life, care of the elderly is gaining the esteem that it deserves. Consultants specialise in the relatively new field of *gerontology*, to study the interrelation of mental, physical and social changes of advanced years. Although some problems can be reasonably expected in older people, their occurrence is by no means inevitable. The majority of people live many happy, healthy years in retirement, providing they can be eased over the hiccups of transient illness or social hardship.

Old age is not a disease entity and it is a mistake to lump all failings under that causative heading. This defeats attempts to correct individual problems, which may be masked by the knock-on effect that manifests as global disturbance.

So the apparently demented old lady may in fact be confused due to overdosage by multiple drug therapy or have a treatable urinary infection. Apathy and lethargy may be signs of anaemia, myxoedema or hypothermia. Loss of weight may signal cancer or depression accompanying bereavement.

Sometimes independence lies in a simple corrective procedure, such as supplying a walking frame, a downstairs commode or a new set of dentures. The detective work of geriatric assessment has to take stock of organic, emotional, mental and social factors, acting on a machine that has been running for a long time and may be showing signs of wear.

The current positive ideals for the specialty of geriatrics has largely emanated from the nursing profession itself, keen to demonstrate just how exacting and rewarding care of the elderly can be. Several clinical courses related to this are available for qualified nurses and many innovative projects are devised and run by nurses who deal with older patients.

All nurses in general training complete a mandatory geriatric module, concentrating on the aims of care for the elderly, both in hospital and the community. With practical work experience in these areas, they will, hopefully, gain some understanding of the full spectrum of progressive care towards rehabilitation. Many young nurses develop a depressing picture of old age, if their only experience is of gravely ill and handicapped elderly in general wards, so it is important that they are aware of the amenities available to aid the independence of the elderly in the community. Figure 11.1 illustrates the range of facilities and personnel which are on hand to support the elderly and their carers when they live at home.

Geriatric unit

A geriatric unit in a general hospital is ideally staffed by a team, trained and committed to the elderly, in understanding their specific needs. A unit should comprise several wards, organised to meet the needs at various level of dependence, aiming to promote an active existence, mobility, continence and self-reliance, as far as can be achieved. Patients progress from acute care, through medium care, then assessment and rehabilitation before returning to the community or going to a continuing care ward. The term of 'medical care for the elderly' may be preferred to 'geriatric medicine', which has a derogatory, unprepossessing connotation.

Reality orientation

The increasing number of the elderly mentally infirm pose a large problem for management. Sometimes they are admitted to a general hospital, to benefit from the full gamut of physical investigations, as well as psychological care. Many are cared for in the community, either by relatives or in part three accommodation or hostels, or in a continuing care ward for psychogeriatric patients in a psychiatric hospital. One important aspect of their

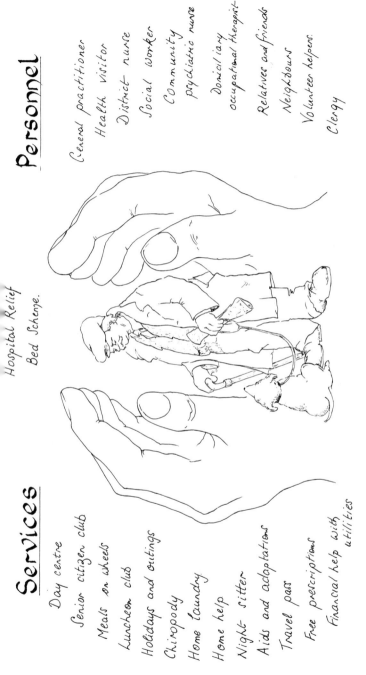

Personnel

General practitioner
Health visitor
District nurse
Social worker
Community
psychiatric nurse
Domiciliary
occupational therapist
Relatives and friends
Neighbours
Volunteer helpers
Clergy

Hospital Relief
Bed Scheme.

Services

Day centre
Senior citizen club
Meals on wheels
Luncheon club
Holidays and outings
Chiropody
Home laundry
Home help
Night sitter
Aids and adaptations
Travel pass
Free prescriptions
Financial help with
utilities

Community Facilities for the Elderly at home.

Fig. 11.1

treatment is called reality orientation, designed to keep the elderly forgetful person in touch with the reality of his environment, especially in time and place. A reality orientation board in the ward clearly states the date and name of the hospital and ward, while the staff reiterate the time of day and try to keep patients abreast of current affairs.

Day hospital and day centre

A day hospital may be attached to a geriatric unit, for patients to be brought in from home, to have a continued programme of nursing care and rehabilitation on a daily basis or for a few sessions a week. This gives the patient a certain degree of independence, while freeing a hospital bed for someone else's use.

Another useful provision is the day centre, organised by the local authority, offering day care of a more social and recreational nature. Not only does it afford a focus of interest for the old person, but it serves the very important additional function of providing a break for the caring relative.

Giving prolonged attention to an elderly person, who may perhaps be truculent, demented, perhaps heavy and incontinent, imposes a considerable strain on even the most conscientious carer. There have been some reports of 'granny bashing', assault on an elderly dependent relative by an overwrought relative, who has finally reacted against the burden of unrelenting responsibility.

One essential service is the hospital *bed relief scheme* of temporary admission for short-term care of an old person, which allows a caring relative to relax or take a holiday. This is also known as *respite* care.

The elderly in the community

It is obvious that a liaison between the primary care service and the hospital authority is vital if the best is to be made of all the available resources to maintain the elderly in the community, to spend a happy, active journey towards the end of life. The idea of community teams for the elderly in the district encompasses the idea of a liaison of services and personnel, to consolidate facilities.

The elderly form a high proportion of the workload of any

district nurse, while there are now some health visitors especially appointed to supervise the aged population in an area. A community psychiatric nurse may be particularly designated to cater for the welfare of the elderly mentally infirm.

Contrary to popular belief, only a tiny proportion of old people require permanent residential care, yet this is often the picture that younger people have of elderly folk, as senile and dependent. Certainly there is a preponderance of elderly people in wards for general medicine and surgery, especially in orthopaedics and ophthalmics, but, after suitable treatment, most can go back home to continue into a fit old age.

In fact, 95 per cent of people beyond retirement age live in the community, either alone or with a spouse, relatives or friends. Any of us could think of the active septuagenarians and octogenarians coping marvellously with their lives. Names quickly spring to mind of those in the older generation who continue to contribute a wealth of wisdom and knowledge to society, in the fields of art, science, medicine, politics and the judiciary. The Third Age University, organised for the retired who wish to expand their education, has been a great success and the Open University has a lot of older students, who are notably very diligent in their studies.

In many more primitive societies the elders are the leaders, rather than western society which dispatches people into retirement at 65—often reluctantly accepted. The average life-expectancy in Britain is 70 for men and 76 for women. In America, the Grey Panther movement is a pressure group, which is making sure that the older generation is not going to be left sitting idle and ignored by their youth-oriented society. There is evidence that British senior citizens are also thinking along the same lines and getting themselves organised to help one another and stimulate public awareness.

In an era when the elderly feel increasingly isolated and vulnerable, it is crucial that the society adopts a caring and considerate attitude, both as individual and corporate responsibility. By extending a friendly, inviting hand, members of a community must help the elderly become involved with general social activities, and be able to recognise and respond to the needs of the elderly around them. This is being done through self-help groups, volunteer agencies and church members. Often it is the younger elderly who are helping the old elderly and, certainly, the newly retired are very useful in this respect and enjoy the involvement themselves. But it is also important that young people are linked with their elderly citizens, to form a communication between these two distant generations.

Of the other 5 per cent of the elderly population, 2½ per cent require some kind of supervised accommodation and it is the merest 2½ per cent that need residential nursing care. The 'old old', those over 85, cause the greatest concern, because with greater frailty they do make an increasing demand on the health and social services.

The elderly in institutions

For those needing continuing care in an institution, the accent is on a homely environment, while retaining ties with the family, friends, pets and the community at large. Residents are encouraged to wear their own clothes and keep personal possessions with them, in an effort to boost morale, to preserve dignity and self-respect, through retaining their individuality.

Thoughtful ideas on nutrition have led to a better diet, with fresh fruit, wholemeal bread and natural juices, rather than the old unappetising food of repetitive mince, mash or sloppy chicken, suitable only for the edentulous masses. A nourishing, wholesome and interesting diet with balanced nutrition obviates the use of vitamin pills and proprietary bowel preparations. It also makes mealtimes a joyful occasion instead of a necessary task to be hurried out of the way.

With the involvement of outsiders, hopefully volunteers, clergy, relatives and school pupils coming to perform their concerts and carol services, the elderly residents are kept in touch with the real world and lead a more enriched life. They may be taken out for a trip to the park or the shops, out for tea or a drink in the pub. In the residential home, many activities can be pursued to stimulate their interest, such as cooking, gardening, music, needlework, current affairs, card games, and gentle exercise classes to improve their mobility.

It is often presumed that relatives 'dump' their elderly dependants into residential accommodation as a social convenience and want no more to do with them. In fact they are usually very willing to help out in a variety of ways, to benefit both their relative and the home in general. It is the enterprising ward sister or warden who makes a welcoming invitation for relatives' help and may perhaps form a relatives' group to encourage and formulate their participation. The local darts team could sponsor for new equipment, or film shows and speakers could be brought in.

As in every area of care, the nurse may find some disparity between the desired ideal and the reality of the work situation. Many nurses are struggling to do their best in horrible old buildings with battered furnishing, yet, time and again, they are praised for their good care, their positive attitude and the happy atmosphere that prevails. People *are* more important than the surroundings. Certainly staff morale is boosted by involvement with a stimulating care programme, which, in more ways than one, reflects well on the patients.

It is encouraging that there is more concern that people live on into an old age of fulfilment, rather than suffer dejection and misery.

Geriatric nursing is not a popular choice of specialty for the younger, newly qualified staff. They prefer the livelier pace of a busy acute area, which continues to carry greater prestige than working with the elderly. But a returning nurse will appreciate having time to spend with each patient and enjoy feeling comfortable doing the basic care which comes easily to her, in a less pressurised environment. Elderly patients will respond warmly to a nurse who has patience and tolerance, with an understanding of their frailties and special needs.

A steep escalation is expected in the elderly population by the year 2000 and beyond. There will be an estimated 9½ million people over retirement age, of which 3 million will be over 75 and around 4000 will be achieving their century.

It is patently untenable for the state to provide for *every* aspect of their welfare, otherwise a situation will develop whereby the half of the community that is working will be occupied in looking after the other half who are children or retired!

Within a positive framework, old people should be helped and encouraged to enjoy the remainder of their life. As more and more people are guided through a young healthy life, care of the elderly poses a considerable national challenge, from both a social and medical standpoint.

Primary care

Primary health care is delivered to people in the community, in their own homes or at a health centre, by members of the primary health care team. This team comprises the general practitioner, district nurse, health visitor, school nurse and possibly a practice nurse helping at the surgery or health centre, and domiciliary midwife.

Other nurse specialists, whose functions are applicable in both the hospital and the community and therefore need to liaise between the two, may be employed to give help and advice in stoma care, breast care, diabetic care, continence or symptom control in terminal illness.

Anyone in the primary care team may also have need to liaise with other community personnel over specific problems, such as community psychiatric nurse, community mental handicap nurse, the school nurse, the social worker, family planning staff and a wide range of voluntary agencies.

Community nursing staff are coordinated by the director of nursing services for the primary and community health care service, and the general practitioner is the medical practitioner to whom they refer. Domiciliary midwives come under the midwifery division and the CPN and CMHN are under the psychiatric division.

Any nurse contemplating any type of work within the community service would be expected to hold a current driving licence and probably to be a car owner.

District nursing

Synonymous with the term 'district nurse' are 'home nurse', 'domiciliary nurse' and 'community nurse', although the latter should not be confused with the community psychiatric nurse, who has an entirely different function.

The district nurse gives nursing care to people in the community, who do not require, or desire, full-time hospitalisation. If the patient and relatives are able to manage at home, then it is cost-effective to save on a hospital bed and have a nurse visit on an occasional basis. This arrangement may also be much appreciated by the patient, in preference to a prolonged stay in hospital away from his family.

A district nurse takes with her the full range of nursing knowledge and skills, to apply in the context of the home. Home nursing is based upon the nursing model of care, comprising assessment of needs, planning and implementation of care plan, followed by evaluation of the outcome. This may involve all basic care, bathing, dressings, injections, stoma care, diabetic management and the care of the postoperative patient.

As a large proportion of her work is continuing care with the elderly, those with long-term conditions or terminal illness, it is crucial that she is able to strike up a good ongoing relationship with the patient and responsible relatives. This is necessary if she is going to fulfil those other important aspects of her role, namely teaching, supporting, advising, counselling and rehabilitation methods, to enable families to function and adapt to the limitations of one individual member.

Heading a small team, the qualified district nurse may be assisted by district enrolled nurses and untrained people, variably called auxiliary nurse, assistant, aid or bath nurse. The Macmillan Home Care Nursing Service and Marie Curie Foundation are able to augment community services and offer practical help and support to relatives, by supplying nurses specifically for the terminally ill person being cared for at home.

All nurses in training undertake a community module, which includes practical experience working with the district nurse and health visitor. For young nurses, who have only ever been used to a tightly structured hospital environment, it is in sharp contrast to see the patient on his own territory and be the visitor for a change. It can be most illuminating to see how nursing must be adapted to meet individual needs in a variety of home surroundings.

It is often erroneously assumed that work on the district would be an easy avenue to return to nursing. This idea is held if district nursing is mistakenly characterised as simply comprising basic nursing tasks. Such an attitude was admirably reflected by a patient who, impressed by the district nurse caring for him in his home, remarked on her efficiency and inquired if she had ever considered being a hospital nurse!

Yet the contemporary district nurse has a highly skilled and responsible role, to evaluate and execute the care plans for her allotted patient caseload. And compared to hospital nurses she works in relative isolation.

A district nursing sister is a registered nurse with two years post-registration experience, who has taken an approved course for nursing in the community and been successful in the examinations. This training is now mandatory for a nurse to practise on the district.

The current college-based course, lasting nine months, leads to the National District Nursing Certificate (NDNCert). It consists of units of theory, together with practice in the community, supervised by a practical work teacher (PWT). The potential district nurse student would require five 'O' levels or the equivalent, and at present all courses are run on a full-time basis, there having been no call for part-time provision.

Enrolled nurses may also take a district nurse training over a period of 16 weeks, but this course is not mandatory, only recommended. RGNs may find some vacancies for part-time work, depending on the employment policy and the availability of full-time staff, perhaps for the twilight shift for a 'back-to-bed' service. There is provision for the ordinary registered nurse to be employed by authorities in a staff nurse capacity on the district, but it is discouraged and should be reserved for those nurses who work while waiting for their course to commence. Any RGN would be accountable to the trained district nurse, so it is rather a waste of a qualified nurse's valuable training.

Both the employment of RGNs and part-time opportunities are becoming a less likely option on the district, since more nurses choose to take the training and to work full-time, thereby taking a full caseload. District nursing does continue to be a popular area of work for married women and there are a small number of men working on the district.

Any nurse wanting to become a district nurse must apply simultaneously for a place on an approved course and employment with an authority prepared to second her, thereby securing payment of fees and having an area for fieldwork. Every national board will have a list of colleges currently running a course in operation for NDNCert.

The earlier Queen's Nurse, holding the QIDNS certificate is licensed to practise on the district. Any qualified district nurse returning after an absence would need to be updated by the employing health authority. This would probably take the form of an induction course, with supervised practice on the district, plus sessions in the hospital, with special reference to lifting technique, use of sterile packs and current practice in nursing and social administration.

Health visiting

The health visitor has a wide range of responsibilities, concerned with the promotion of health and prevention of physical, mental and social illness. Her role involves advice, counselling, support and health education for all sections of the community: help aimed at getting people to stand on their own feet and be in control of their lives. She is well placed to call on the resources and personnel, both voluntary and statutory, who can add their contribution to aid vulnerable people.

Traditionally, a major component of the work of the health visitor relates to child health, to the under-fives, and to support of new mothers adjusting to their unfamiliar role. This comprises antenatal classes, home visits to the expectant mother and an obligation to visit when the mother and child have been discharged from maternity care. Follow-up of new families depends on their subsequent need, apart from the periodic developmental assessments and immunisation programme. Many mothers attend the child health clinic on an informal basis and will ask the health visitor if they are concerned about any particular aspect of the child's progress.

Also within the province of the health visitor comes supervision of people with long-term illness, the recently bereaved, those with social problems and patients recently discharged from hospital. With the increasing move to maintain handicapped and disabled people in the community, the health visitor is expected to offer her expertise to these people and their families.

Some districts now employ a health visitor with the precise responsibility of monitoring the increasing number of elderly living in the community, many very old and frail who manage to live alone. Preventive surveillance would detect any insidious problems that are amenable to treatment, which the old person has dismissed as being due to old age. The service may be organised on a team basis, incorporating the skills of the district nurse, the health visitor and the community psychiatric nurse, all working closely with the community and the hospital services.

The health visitor has a unique function, being fundamentally the prime agent for prevention and positive health counselling within the community. She is an impartial point of contact, and is often the only professional worker to visit the home of some needy clients on a regular basis.

By understanding and evaluating the special health-related social needs of her particular community, the health visitor modifies her practice locally. She may be concerned with the needs of homeless, immigrant or gypsy families, pregnant teenagers or families under hardship from unemployment or inadequate housing. The health visitor can be instrumental in the formation of support groups: for mothers in their postnatal period; for captive mothers to escape from an isolated existence; or for parents to share their grief if their child has died, as in sudden infant death syndrome (SIDS), or 'cot death'.

Most health visitors are now attached to a general practitioner or group practice and work with patients from that list, although some may be assigned to a geographical area. The idea of an 'at-risk register' is useful to highlight special groups of people requiring extra support and attention, such as child abuse or battered wives, or those with an alcohol or drug problem.

Health visitor training is open to registered nurses with certified obstetric experience, plus five 'O' levels or the equivalent. The post-registration college-based course lasts for one year, although there are several colleges which operate a part-time course over a two-year period. The training includes lectures, discussions and practical experience under the guidance of a fieldwork teacher for the academic year, followed by final examinations and three months supervised practice with a small caseload.

Every national board has a list of colleges offering health visitor training. A prospective health visitor student would need to apply simultaneously to a college to gain a place on the course and a health authority for secondment. If a returning nurse does not have the required obstetric experience, this can usually be arranged within the health district.

Those returning to health visiting would need a comprehensive updating of their work initially, and are kept abreast of changes by subsequent refresher courses.

Practice nursing

With the general practitioner as the prime source of contact for all medical, and many social, problems there are a number of ways in which the nurse can assist the doctor with a variety of duties.

A practice nurse can relieve a doctor of routine tasks, such as taking temperatures, pulse and blood pressures, testing urine, taking swabs, ear syringing, injections and dressings. She can help with patients who require physical examination and then follow on with patient education, perhaps explaining how to instil eye drops or take suppositories. Her role extends to counselling and health advice, talking about diet or breast examination, handing out education leaflets, all of which is valuable preventive work.

Patients occasionally want to seek advice but do not necessarily need a medical consultation, so if a nurse is available she can absorb or deflect many inquiries. Frequently patients are reassured that they can visit or telephone the nurse, without having to 'worry the busy doctor'. General practitioners do get bogged down with, and often irritated by, what they consider is the 'trivia' of general practice, not essentially requiring a doctor's expertise.

The young wife comes out with a prescription for valium, when the root cause of her anxiety is that her husband may have been made redundant. A mother may simply want to ask about her child's rash, or be concerned about his bowel motions, or whether his cut leg is worthy of a visit to casualty. Another wants to seek reassurance about her menstrual cycle or back pain, or to have a blood pressure check in the case of headaches. Many minor ailments conceal an underlying social or emotional problem, and a nurse can give that precious commodity of 'time', to allow the patient to talk and off-load his anxiety. Of course, whenever there is doubt the nurse must refer patients to the general practitioner.

An extension of this role is the development on the American lines of a nurse practitioner, who assumes a more comprehensive set of duties within the general practice, and frequently proves a popular option for patients.

As the average general practitioner consultation takes six minutes, there may certainly be room to develop the role of nurses working in general practice, especially with the increasing emphasis on preventive health and patient education towards self-care.

The RCN Society of Primary Health Care Nursing could give further information about the role of the nurse in general practice as it is currently applied.

School nursing

The school nurse is responsible for the supervision of health care of schoolchildren, beyond the age of five until they leave school. Her role includes health surveys with comprehensive medical assessments and screening procedures to check normal development and spot any irregularities. She is concerned with vision and hearing, height and weight, hygiene checks and the immunisation programme.

The role of the school nurse encompasses health education to pupils and counselling over emotional or behavioural difficulties, in conjunction with other members of the primary care team, teachers and parents. The periodic reviews at school may be the only form of health checks routinely provided for the developing child, unless illness brings him into contact with the general practitioner.

With the increasing integration of handicapped children into normal schools, the nurse must be familiar with the special needs of children who have a variety of disabilities through mental and physical handicap.

A 12-week college-based course with supervised practical experience prepares the registered nurse or sick children's nurse for the School Nurse Certificate.

Although this training is not yet a mandatory requirement to employment as a school nurse, primary care authorities are keen to second their nurses for a course, to enable them to pursue their role to its fullest capacity.

The school nurse is concerned with the ongoing surveillance of the school age population and will be employed to cover several schools in one geographical location.

Her role must not be confused with the welfare assistant working in a particular school for the day-to-day supervision of children on the premises. A welfare assistant is often mistakenly called the 'nurse' because she copes with first aid, sudden illness, and gives daytime medication, but she is employed by the education authority. Although it is advantageous for her to be a nurse, her function does not equate with that of the school nurse in the primary health service.

The school nurse is ideally employed in a full-time capacity, although there may be some part-time posts available. A full-timer cannot necessarily expect to work school hours with the long school holidays free, although obviously most of her work is concentrated during term time.

A welfare assistant does work school hours and has time off in the holidays, so this is an ideal job for a woman with children of her own at school. There is an increasing demand for welfare assistants to help in nursery units and schools where there are a lot of handicapped children, needing toileting and help with calipers.

Carers in the community

No section on primary care would be complete without mention of the vital role played by the army of 'invisible angels', the stoic, unsung, unpaid—and often unrecognised—carers in the community. Much attention has recently been focused on these relatives and companions who make an inestimable contribution to maintain the elderly, sick, frail and handicapped in homely surroundings and in the bosom of their family.

By devoting much of their time and energy to the foremost needs of a dependent relative, carers sacrifice their own career prospects, are often denied the chance to earn a wage and accrue a pension, as well as losing touch with friends and social pursuits. An invalid care allowance, as compensation for giving up a full-time job, is only payable to a male or *single* female carer. Any woman who is married or cohabiting is presumed to be staying at home anyway and not eligible for that allowance. This effectively discounts three-quarters of all carers, something like 78 000 married women, devoted to round-the-clock nursing and supervision, cook, cleaner and companion to a dependent relative.

The caring person may herself be ailing and retired, perhaps a 70-year-old lady looking after her 95-year-old father. Alternatively, a ten-year-old schoolboy may be assuming a lot of household duties, when managing with a mother who has multiple sclerosis. Young families may move to a larger house with the express intention of accommodating a single elderly parent or handicapped child, which in itself has tremendous implications for family relationships and finances. Lone carers are imprisoned by the fearful responsibility of leaving a demented relative, who may be a danger to himself or the property.

Carers are caught in a dilemma and consequently experience ambivalence about their situation. While accepting that they are doing the right thing for their loved one, they are denied much of their own full life. Many struggle on in isolation, coping with an increasingly difficult set of circumstances. Theirs is a job with no off-duty hours or days, no holiday to look forward to, and perhaps no one to relieve them of the total burden of physical and emotional responsibility.

There are times when I feel so tired and fed up, I haven't been able to take a holiday for eight years. I've not had much of a life of my own, if ever I make plans to go out, Dad gets ill. Besides I couldn't trust him with the fire and gas stove and his cigarettes. He treats me like a little girl and takes everything I do for granted. Sometimes, I wish it would all end, but then I feel so guilty.

The final toll may result in a breakdown of the relationship of the carer with their relative, resulting in abuse, or breakdown of the family, resulting in marital discord. The principal carer may herself become a victim of mental or physical overload with the intolerable strain of unrelenting responsibility.

Because the assistance is so greatly valued, indeed relied upon, and the carer's ultimate health is of concern, it behoves the primary care team to offer help and guidance in any possible way they can. This might include referral to useful agencies and voluntary services, provision of nursing care, a night sitter, a hospital short-term admission, practical advice on lifting and continence, as well as interpretation of the social benefits available. One enterprising idea is to amalgamate this instruction and information into a useful course for carers, involving a wide range of professionals to offer their expertise.

Any situation which poses continuing care in the community must be the joint responsibility between the relative, the health service and social service, primarily with the members of the community health care team.

It is estimated that if only 1 per cent of the carers withdrew from their role, then community services would be required to increase their expenditure by an astounding 20 per cent to care for dependent people in the community.

Care of sick children

Within the space of three generations, the knowledge accrued about child development and maternal attachment has completely revolutionised attitudes to paediatric care.

Grandmothers of today would hardly equate their horrifyingly traumatic hospital experiences with the comfort, fun and liberty that their grandchildren are ideally likely to encounter.

Quite obviously the dramatic alteration in disease patterns and treatments has made a huge contribution to these changes. Contagious diseases no longer pose a threat to the lives of children who are well-nourished and in good health. Antibiotics get rid of those infections which used to lead to chronic incapacitating conditions, such as heart valve disease, kidney failure, meningitis or deafness. This obviates those earlier rigorous isolation measures, found to be so emotionally damaging to a child, whose care was surrendered to white-clad attendants, with only infrequent visits allowed by the parents.

Protracted conservative treatments in orthopaedics, which often required months or years in a distant hospital, have fallen into disfavour, because the social and psychological disruption conflicts with the beneficial effects. Surgery has played an increasing part particularly in this specialty.

Tuberculosis, polio and diphtheria are childhood diseases that have been banished into history—with an active immunisation programme to ensure that they stay there!

Rigorous routine checks on the infant at birth, in health clinics and at school, will detect and correct abnormalities at an early stage, for example, club foot, congenital dislocated hip (CDH), cleft palate and heart defects.

Any child born with a mental or physical handicap is helped from the outset to maximise his potential, while parents are given full support to enable them to care for him in a family setting.

Paediatric units have a different environment, altered concepts of care and are involved in advanced and enterprising methods of treatment. With improved anaesthetics, superior surgical techniques and intensive postoperative care, doctors push back the frontiers to make courageous efforts to improve the lives of children who, in earlier times, would never have had any chance of survival.

It is not unusual to see heroic surgery in spina bifida, the correction of scoliosis using a metal rod insertion, and heart, kidney or liver transplants. Similarly, tremendous progress has been made with children who have malignant conditions, those with tumours are subject to vigorous treatment programmes, and leukaemia sufferers can have a reasonable life expectancy. Specialties such as these are frequently restricted to a regional unit, which admits children from all over the country, as well as the local region. Centres of excellence are often found in teaching hospitals, providing care for heart surgery or oncology, two rapidly expanding fields.

As ever-younger preterm babies are being offered hope for survival, aided by an abundance of sophisticated equipment, *neonatology* has become a subspecialty within the paediatric field. The clinical course for special baby care is a popular post-basic option for both paediatric nurses and midwives.

From the social side of medicine, we witness children who have been involved in solvent abuse, or who are victims of sexual abuse, or 'non-accidental injury', which supersedes the emotive and accusatory term of 'battered baby syndrome'.

In a society where there is a fairly high incidence of divorce, children who come from broken homes or one-parent families may have additional practical and emotional difficulties when they are admitted to hospital.

So the nurse employed in a modern paediatric setting may find the work emotionally and physically demanding. On the one hand there are the brief admissions and rapid discharges adding to the workload. On the other hand she is faced with the intensive care of children undergoing critical surgery or nursing those who are gravely ill with long-term illness.

The nurse is no longer the person who *takes over* the care of a child, but finds herself as a member of the team, in which the parents' contribution is vital.

Children in hospital

Nowadays, parents are encouraged to remain with children who need to be admitted to hospital and to share in the care wherever possible. Nurses who are new to this philosophy may feel very threatened that their own role has been usurped by a capable mother. It will take some readjustment of ideas, to consider what is in the best interests of the young patient in their charge, who is in an alien situation.

It is desirable that mothers stay with children under the age of five, which is the most vulnerable stage as regards separation (see Fig. 11.2). Many hospitals now provide facilities for mothers to 'room in' with babies and infants, which is conducive to continuation of breast feeding. In a makeshift situation, mother is given a fold-up bed in the child's cubicle, or in long-stay situations there may be a separate mothers' home or bed and breakfast accommodation provided near the hospital. It is always useful if some neutral territory is available, like a communal sitting room or cafeteria, where mothers may relax away from the ward in the company of other adults. Parents are not charged to accompany their child in hospital but do pay for meals which are usually bought in the staff canteen.

Mothers can contribute to any care in which they feel able, such as giving feeds, bathing, dressing or playing with her child

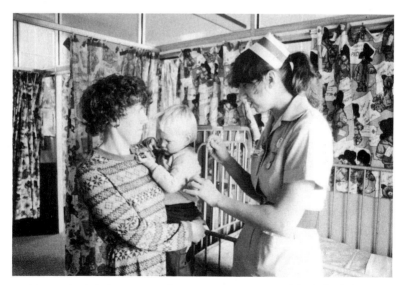

Fig. 11.2 It is important that parents can stay with their children in hospital. (Reproduced by courtesy of NAWCH; photo by Michael Hardy.)

or accompanying him to departments. After adequate instruction, some mothers feel confident to undertake tube feeding of their tiny premature baby, while supervised, in the special care baby unit. But it must also be appreciated that parents often feel terrorstruck at handling their very sick child.

While wholeheartedly endorsing the policy that mothers stay with their ill child, it should be remembered that this may present different kinds of problems if there are siblings at home who also need their mother. These children may be traumatised by their mother's continued absence and apparent over-indulgence of one child. So visiting by all members of the family is to be encouraged, especially brothers and sisters who want to see what the mystery is all about.

When older children are admitted to hospital, the ideal arrangement is for unrestricted visiting. This allows parents to visit at any time of the day or night, when the child needs them most, for example immediately before and after surgery or to accompany them to a special investigation.

Flexible visiting means that visitors—parents, siblings, relatives, friends—are welcome at any time during the day, providing it doesn't interfere with meals, treatments or school schedule. Granny may prefer to travel on the bus in the afternoon, rather than in the evening or father may visit in the morning if he is on night work.

Visits can be as long or as short as necessary and parents can leave when a child is contented or sleepy—a complete reversal of the grim days of stringent visiting hours, when distraught mothers had their screaming children plucked from their skirts, as the bell rang on the dot of seven!

Special mention must be made here of the National Association for the Welfare of Children in Hospital (NAWCH), who have waged an unerring campaign to press for improved facilities and conditions for hospitalised children and their parents. The situation is far from ideal and they hope to see the universal acceptance and adoption of modern philosophies of the care of children in hospital (see Figures 11.3 and 11.4).

These days children are prepared in advance for hospital visits by a selection of useful books and leaflets designed for their comprehension at an early age. Hospitalisation should be, within its limits, a happy experience for all concerned.

It is strongly recommended that children be nursed on wards

NAWCH CHARTER

FOR CHILDREN IN HOSPITAL

1

Children shall be admitted to hospital only if the care they require
cannot be equally well provided at home or on a day basis.

2

Children in hospital shall have the right to have their parents with
them at all times provided this is in the best interest of the child.
Accommodation should therefore be offered to all parents, and
they should be helped and encouraged to stay. In order to share
in the care of their child, parents should be fully informed about
ward routine and their active participation encouraged.

3

Children and/or their parents shall have the right to information
appropriate to age and understanding.

4

Children and/or their parents shall have the right to informed
participation in all decisions involving their health care.
Every child shall be protected from unnecessary
medical treatment and steps taken to mitigate
physical or emotional distress.

5

Children shall be treated with tact and understanding and at all times
their privacy shall be respected.

6

Children shall enjoy the care of appropriately trained staff, fully aware
of the physical and emotional needs of each age group.

7

Children shall be able to wear their own clothes and have their own
personal possessions.

8

Children shall be cared for with other children of the same age group.

9

Children shall be in an environment furnished and equipped to meet
their requirements, and which conforms to recognised standards
of safety and supervision.

10

Children shall have full opportunity for play, recreation and education
suited to their age and condition.

NAWCH, National Association for the Welfare of Children in Hospital
Argyle House, 29-31 Euston Road, London, NW1 2SD. Telephone 01-833 2041
Published November 1984

Fig. 11.3 NAWCH charter for children in hospital.

Parents' role

Mothers and fathers are encouraged to participate in the general nursing of their children. This will include bathing and dressing, feeding, toilet training (if still required). You will only be asked to help with the more detailed care at the discretion of the doctor or ward sister.

Unless your child is confined to the cubicle for medical reasons we hope you and your child will take part in the activities in the ward.

Nursing and medical staff are available to give advice and help.

Play

Opportunity for play throughout your child's stay in hospital contributes to his wellbeing.

The hospital play leader and her assistants set up play activities in the ward and we hope that you and your child will take part.

Schoolwork

During term times a school teacher provides educational facilities for children who are of school age and who are well enough to participate. Lessons are held in the mornings only.

Accommodation

The parent shares a cubicle with his/her child. Each cubicle has a wash basin and toilet. Mother/father is responsible for making his/her own bed, general tidiness of the cubicle and adjoining wash basin and toilet.

A bathroom and toilet is available at the end of the ward.

A sitting room for parents is on Chaucer Ward. Television is available here.

Meals and snacks

1. Meals may be taken in the staff dining room, please obtain a pass from sister, or Jane Tibble, the receptionist for parents.

Breakfast 08.00–09.00 h
Lunch 12–14.00 h
Supper 18.30–20.00 h

Fig. 11.4 Notes for the guidance of parents at Northwick Park Hospital, Harrow. (Reproduced by kind permission of Nursing Times where they were published on February 1, 1979.)

2. Beverages (tea, coffee), can be made in the kitchenette at the end of the ward, and of course you are expected to wash up and leave the kitchenette tidy. Please bring your own tea and coffee. Milk and hot water are supplied free.

No dishes/cutlery are to be kept in the cubicles.

3. The tea bar in outpatients department is open from 09.30–17.00 h Monday to Friday, and may be used by parents and visitors.

There is also a snack vending machine in the accident and emergency department.

Other facilities

A public telephone is available in the ward.

In the shopping square (off the main internal street, on Level 4) there is a hairdresser, a bank (Lloyds), a general shop (run by the League of Friends selling magazines, newspapers, tobacco, gifts, tea, coffee) and a library.

The general shop is open in the evenings and at weekends, as well as during the day.

Outside the main lifts (by the wards) on Level 4 there is a fruit and flower (plus other commodities) shop. This is also open in the evenings and at weekends.

Halfway along the main internal street, Level 4, is a multi-denominational chapel.

Requirements for parents living in

Day and night clothes.

As there are no laundry facilities, clothes should be sent home for washing.

Toilet requisites.

Knitting, sewing, reading material or other suitable hobbies.

Valuables or large amounts of money should not be brought to the hospital, as liability cannot be accepted by the hospital.

SMOKING IS NOT PERMITTED IN CUBICLES OR WARD AREAS.

If you have any queries or problems between 9 and 4pm ask for Jane, the family receptionist.

If you have problems with accommodation for your other children perhaps while father is at work, please let us know.

organised specifically for child patients and they should be cared for either by, or under the direction of, trained paediatric nurses. The idea of admitting children to specialist adult wards is expressly discouraged but can still be found in areas like ENT and burns.

A children's ward should be informal, flexible, cheerfully decorated and geared to the needs of young patients—it should not be expected to stay in apple-pie order. There should be a plentiful supply of toys and stimulating activities, since play has been recognised as a vital component in every child's development.

A *play leader* and nursery nurses organise constructive activities for young children, while older children continue their school studies under the guidance of a hospital teacher. Groups of ambulant children gather in the playroom, while a bedbound patient is set some absorbing task. It is quite a remarkable balancing act to see a child in traction busy doing a painting or stirring a cake!

A variety of other staff are employed in an attempt to reduce the stress of hospitalisation for all members of the family. The social worker can offer support and advice of a practical and emotional nature.

Other helpers may be used to cover the multitude of sundry tasks that appear on any paediatric ward, from reading a child a story, helping with a puzzle, comforting a worried mother to putting up Christmas decorations. Depending on local policy, this may be attributed to a ward clerk, a family receptionist, a ward granny or a voluntary helper.

As a general policy, periods in hospital for children are kept as short as possible to minimise the disruption of home life, normal schooling and local friendships. The average length of stay for a child in 1959 was 15 days, which by 1979 had been reduced to a mere three days.

Day surgery has become increasingly popular for minor operations on children, for example circumcision, herniorrhaphy or insertion of grommets. Many investigations, assessments and treatments may be conducted on an outpatient basis, either in a clinic or on the paediatric ward. Some families may need to make frequent visits to the ward for ongoing support from the staff over some chronic condition, in cases of leukaemia, asthma, epilepsy or juvenile arthritic conditions.

It is just this kind of ease of communication and access to professional staff that exemplifies the new emphasis in paediatrics on family-centred care and the team approach. The nurse must consider each child in the context of his family and parental involvement. It is a formidable position, needing constant adjustment between two roles, on the one hand maintaining a low profile and supporting a mother, and at the next moment taking over direct care of the child when the mother has to leave.

The wider role of the paediatric nurse involves support and education for the whole family, as well as care for the child patient. This is something that the mature, returning nurse will understand well. The needs of a mother who is constantly with her sick child must be met by allowing her a welcome break to escape from the stress and boredom of the situation, while knowing her child is well supervised.

Training

RSCN/RGN is taken as a basic combined training in three years eight months. The post-registration course for RGNs lasts for 13 months, provided that the nurse has had paediatric experience during her training.

The nursing model of care works well in the paediatric situation, with care tailored to the specific needs of each child and his parents. It is desirable that a child builds a relationship with a limited number of people, so is assigned to his 'special' nurse, who will be responsible for the full spectrum of care.

Paediatric nurse training includes normal development of the child and assessments of progress, which can be readily observed in a community module working alongside a health visitor or school nurse.

As positive treatment for handicapped children forms a large part of paediatric nursing, it is important that learners gain a deeper knowledge and understanding of their special needs.

The returning nurse may find she has much to offer in a paediatric setting, and certainly the presence of a mature nurse would be especially welcomed by the mothers. However, women who have children of their own may find it unduly distressing to work with seriously ill children and their families. Being in a position where you may identify closely with the family can lead unwittingly to over-involvement.

What you gain in empathy, you may lose in detachment.

Midwifery

The returning nurse with recent experience of the maternity service will have noticed tremendous changes within this specialty. Modern obstetrics has at its disposal an ever-increasing array of technical facilities, to ensure the safety of mother and baby during pregnancy and childbirth.

Few people could claim to be immune to the media hype which fuels the emotive debate between high-tech births versus natural methods. Powerful arguments are lobbed from both within the profession and by involved parties outside, not least of all the mothers on the receiving end.

Advocates of high-tech, who favour scientific input, point to improvement in maternal and perinatal mortality rates as conclusive proof of benefit. Converse argument looks to the quality of the experience of childbirth and is concerned that intervention of the natural process is all too readily assumed, citing enthusiasm for instrumental delivery, near-routine episiotomy, socially convenient induction and indiscriminate monitoring.

Complaints are levelled at the 'conveyor belt system' of obstetrics, which can too easily disregard the individual, having the effect of debasing and depersonalising the unique experience of childbirth.

In particular, visits to the antenatal clinic have been held in the spotlight, where appointments are brief and impersonal and substantial delays in discomfort are commonplace. While antenatal supervision has been acknowledged as a crucial factor in the happy outcome of a pregnancy, shoddy handling is irksome and may effectively drive patients from this important service. Enlightened clinics have devised a realistic appointments system, provide attractive waiting areas, refreshments and toys, or possibly a crèche for accompanying children.

The 'hospital versus home' debate is an extension of high-tech versus natural birth, and both continue unabated. Here is modern medicine clashing with traditional values.

With obvious advantages and disadvantages to each, the conclusion boils down to what is right for each individual family, in terms of personal preference and obstetric requirements. Perhaps the crucial word 'choice' is what underpins the whole controversy. A well-informed mother would like to have some say in the way that the birth of her child is conducted and to be consulted over where she is delivered, the position she adopts, the choice of analgesia and infant feeding.

The National Childbirth Trust (NCT) is a charity which gives active support and information to prospective parents, to educate them about the physiology of childbirth and medical options. They conduct antenatal classes, give postnatal support and counselling about baby feeding. This provides a much-needed link for today's mothers, whose experience of maternity matters is severely limited in this nuclear family society.

The Association for Improvement in Maternity Services (AIMS) is a pressure group concerned with bringing improvements in maternity care.

The midwife balances very delicately in her role. As advocate of the patient, it is important that she considers the latter's desires. Yet she is constrained by the policies of the hospital and the decisions of the doctor, many of whom are less than sympathetic to mothers who bring in their shopping list of maternity requests.

A compromise has to be reached. The woman must be allowed an enjoyable birth close to her specification, while ensuring that, at no time, does this jeopardise the safety of herself or her child.

The vast majority of deliveries do take place in hospital, where all the emergency facilities and specialist staff are at hand. Hospitals are attempting to minimise the stark, antiseptic atmosphere by providing homely side rooms, where the mother may remain throughout her labour and deliver in a normal bed.

Unless monitoring is medically indicated, mothers are permitted to walk freely during the first stage of labour. Borning beds and birthing chairs are increasingly made available to allow a woman to assume an upright position for delivery.

Something like 90 per cent of fathers attend the birth of their child and are generally thrilled to share the experience with their wife. Enlightened units also permit 'significant others', like the mother or friend or cohabitee to join a single woman who is giving birth.

Certain attention has recently been focused on the importance of preconceptual care, which aims to get both partners fully fit and healthy before embarking upon a pregnancy.

The expansion of the fertility aid programme in a wide variety of directions, imposes extra demands on midwives and calls for additional skills and training.

The 'breast is best' campaign has paid dividends by encouraging mothers to make an enthusiastic start in hospital, although many fail to continue breastfeeding once they are back at home if unsupported by a professional.

Home deliveries are few and far between. This has eroded the role of the community midwife, robbed of the satisfaction of sharing the ultimate moment of birth with the family she has prepared over the months.

A good compromise for both mother and midwife is the *domino scheme* (domino stands for 'domiciliary midwife in and out'). The midwife and doctor share antenatal care but the birth is conducted in hospital by the community midwife, who also attends to postnatal care. A domino mother may leave hospital after six hours providing all is well. She will have had the satisfaction of continuous care by one person throughout her pregnancy and confinement.

A community midwife may also be involved with a general practitioner obstetric unit in a hospital, which allows for continuity of care. Her other task is to supervise postnatal care of mothers on planned early discharge (48-hour transfer).

Midwives have generally been concerned over the progressive erosion of their autonomy as practitioners in their own right, fearing they will become maternity nurses at the behest of obstetricians. One group of midwives keen to reaffirm the need for midwifery to provide a complete service to the mother and child have organised themselves to become the Association of Radical Midwives (ARM).

Some independent midwives have set up practice on a private basis, giving a total maternity service to the paying client.

Training

The modern midwifery student has to incorporate a vast body of knowledge, as well as skills related to patient care geared to sophisticated equipment and contemporary methods: ultrasound, partogram, fetal monitoring, epidural anaesthesia, amniocentesis, psychoprophylaxis.

Neonatal care in a special care baby unit (SCBU), previously premature baby unit (PBU), continues to push back the limits of viability. As tiny babies from a 23-week pregnancy struggle to survive, the profound question is begged, can anyone born under 28 weeks gestation still continue to be called an abortion, as the law now stands?

The responsibilities previously belonging to the Central Midwives Boards (CMB) have now been passed to the central body of the UKCC and national boards.

The basic midwifery training is three years for direct entrants and 18 months for a registered general nurse (RGN). There is no longer any reduction in training for any nurse on other parts of the register or roll.

The need for an extended period of midwifery training had been evident for some time but the impetus for its introduction came in to comply with the EEC Midwives' Directives. Midwifery training provides wide experience in all relevant hospital departments, antenatal and postnatal care, labour ward, special care baby unit, together with community experience to prepare for domiciliary care and parent education.

A single period of training supersedes the previous two-part system, which proved a waste of training resources when so many nurses only took part one to gain experience and a useful qualification for their career enhancement, but had no intention of taking part two to practise midwifery.

As a result of the Sex Discrimination Act, men have been able to train as midwives at a limited number of schools.

All nurses in general nurse training are required to have an obstetric allocation, to gain experience in maternity care and nursing the newborn.

An Advanced Diploma of Midwifery (ADM) is available to those who wish to study more deeply in this specialty, and the ADM is a prerequisite to midwifery teaching.

Every midwife is required to take mandatory refresher courses on a regular basis to legally continue in practice. A returning midwife would need to consult the UKCC about if and how she could return to practice, and to update her experience. The Royal College of Midwives would also be a useful contact for this information.

Mental illness

The medical, social and legal reforms of the 20th century have been directed towards dispelling the fearful and fallacious notions of mental illness that had been propounded over previous centuries. Strange, incomprehensible behaviour had been attributed to witchcraft, demonic possession, evil spirits or phases of the moon, from where the word 'lunatic' is derived.

While managing to reject sorcery on an intellectual level, it is harder to shake off those primeval fears of the unknown and bizarre. Fighting the stigma attached to mental illness has been an uphill struggle. The disturbed person has traditionally been banished from the community which he may hurt, taint or contaminate, dispatched to custodial care in a place of isolation.

The battle for the mind has been a double-edged attack. Greater understanding of psychological and sociological processes was one important step forward in the search for positive modes of treatment. The other aim was to achieve greater tolerance for the ill person, to enable him to be integrated back into a society that would accept him. It did eventually become recognised that mental disorders were usually of a temporary or remitting nature, amenable to treatment.

In 1930, people were permitted to enter a mental hospital to seek treatment on a voluntary basis, as opposed to the old loss of liberty and incarceration imposed by being 'certified' or 'committed'.

There can be no doubt that the development of the psychotrophic drugs in the 1950s, and their subsequent expansion onto the market, dramatically altered the nature and prognosis of mental illness. The phenothiazine group of major tranquillisers, such as chlorpromazine (Largactil), had an enormous impact on the control of the severe disorders of schizophrenia and manic-depressive psychosis. Antidepressants, such as amitriptyline (Tryptizol) and imipramine (Tofranil), and anxiolytic drugs, such as diazepam (Valium) and chlordiazepoxide (Librium), have placed many minor psychiatric disorders within the scope of the general practitioner.

It is worth mentioning that the over-liberal and injudicious administration of these minor tranquillisers is now being scrutinised, especially as many have been shown to be addictive with prolonged use. Thirty years on, there is a swing away from the dangerous maxim of 'a pill for every ill', particularly when the root cause is often of social origin.

Also in the 1950s new ideas with the therapeutic community concept and behavioural techniques were increasingly gaining acceptance. Improved treatment methods and positive aims of rehabilitation heralded a new era in the care for the mentally ill, which was reflected in the Mental Health Act of 1959.

There was a grand reappraisal of the legislation relating to mental health across the board. One very important alteration was to enable patients to enter a mental hospital in an 'informal' status, to retain their civil rights, in the same way as people enter a general hospital for physical treatment.

The vast majority of mental hospital patients are now admitted informally, although there are 'sections' within the Act to make provision for compulsory admission when required.

Tolerance and understanding towards the mentally ill by the public has been assisted by media exposure of the subject in a matter-of-fact way. Depression, anxiety and phobias are well known and psychiatric drugs are household names. It is common knowledge that mental illness is not selective, that it can affect anybody, and indeed does occur in one in eight women and one in 14 men sometime in their lives—but it is usually transient and can be treated.

Certainly mental disorder has been made acceptable by the application of new terminology. The use of the term 'psychiatry' has sanitised and intellectualised the specialty, although it is worth noting that we still train the registered *mental* nurse (RMN) and the enrolled nurse (*mental*), EN(M).

'Breakdown', 'neurosis', 'psychiatric problem' is infinitely preferable to 'insanity', 'madness' or 'lunacy'. Recovery is implicit in the first words, as is the temporary or mild nature of the disorder, while the last three indicate a permanent and irretrievable derangement of the mind.

The National Association for Mental Health (MIND) is a voluntary organisation which presses for improvements in the statutory health services and is interested in the legal rights of patients and their general welfare, especially community help.

The 'open-door policy' of the 1960s soon became known disparagingly as the 'revolving door', as patients made frequent, repeated admissions, if they were unable to get to grips with the outside world. Of course, even sharp, short visits are better than the unreal life of an institution, but it was evident that some solution was required to give support and continued care within the community. For precisely this purpose, the community psychiatric nursing service was developed and it has grown to provide a substantial part of the current mental health programme.

Facilities for treatment are now available in psychiatric units attached to general hospitals, ideally staffed by those trained in mental nursing. Although it is hoped that all acute care could be given in these units or contained within the community, there are many aspects of psychiatric work which need long-term care, not least in the elderly population. Future aims are that the old large forbidding mental institutions, mostly relics of the Victorian age, will be closed for ever. Although most have been able to make a substantial reduction in their bed complement, it must be remembered that the word 'asylum'—meaning 'a place of refuge'—should have a respected place in psychiatric care.

Whereas the community psychiatric service has become well established, there has not been a comparable increase in accommodation suitable to house ex-patients who are unable to make their own arrangements. Likewise, employment may also pose a problem for the discharged mentally ill at a time of high unemployment and economic recession. There is considerable concern that patients are being discharged without supervision, to live as vagrants wandering the streets and sleeping rough.

Other areas of psychiatric care in which the nurse may work are alcoholism, drug abuse, psychosexual counselling and forensic psychiatry. The latter refers to the situation where mental disorder coincides with criminal behaviour and the place of treatment and type of care has always been rather contentious: should it be hospital, treatment and nursing care or prison, punishment and warders?

Where treatment seems possible, yet containment is necessary in the interests of the public, an intermediate solution has been arranged. Each regional health authority is required to provide a *secure unit*, which is a locked area with a high staff/patient ratio. A special allowance is payable to staff working in a secure unit or special hospital (such as Broadmoor), in addition to the psychiatric lead, payable to all nurses working in the field of mental health.

Among changes brought about by the Mental Health Act of 1983, registered mental nurses have been invested with a responsibility unique within the nursing profession. Psychiatric nurses have a holding power of not more than six hours, to detain an informal patient who might, if allowed to leave hospital, be a danger to himself or others.

Training

Mental nurse training is geared to modern ideas in psychiatry, psychology and sociology. Physical treatments are now limited to electroconvulsive therapy (ECT) and drug therapy, while more emphasis is placed upon psychosocial and interactive skills, behaviour modification, group therapy, rehabilitation and community care. The use of diagnostic labelling is discouraged throughout psychiatric practice.

The nurse has become a key therapeutic figure in the field of interpersonal relationships, although her role overlaps and intertwines with other members of the mental health team, namely psychiatrist, psychologist, occupational therapist, social worker and, in the community, general practitioner, health visitor, district nurse.

Psychiatric learners have a secondment to a general hospital for experience in general nursing care and this is especially valuable for their work with the elderly mentally ill. This area of care, particularly the demented patients, will figure largely in the future with the growth of the elderly population, and falls within the province of both the general and psychiatric nurse, both in hospital and in the community.

Nurses in general training have a psychiatric secondment to gain understanding of mental illness and related nursing care within this specialty. Seeing 'how the other half live' is a valuable experience for both sets of learners. This mutual overlap of learners should demonstrate how false it is to demarcate between physical and emotional needs and care within the individual.

In a community module within their training, mental nurses learn about social services and community facilities. They are likely to work alongside a *community psychiatric nurse* (CPN) and may visit a day hospital, a day centre and a residential hostel.

The way in which mental nurses are taught should diverge from the traditional teaching methods of chalk-and-talk lecturing, to include some experiental learning. By working in groups, being involved in discussions, they examine group dynamics, their own feelings and how they interact with colleagues. Experience in role play provides the basis of understanding how patients will feel and react.

During the training course, which is three years for RMN, two years for EN(M) and 18 months post-registration, the learner has four ward-based practical assessments similar to those for the general training.

A final national statutory qualifying examination on completion of the course, consists of an essay question paper and an objective paper of multiple choice questions.

There is currently only one basic combined course for RGN/ RMN and a few basic RMN courses which also combine with a degree, usually in social sciences.

Further opportunities in advance training for RMNs lie in many directions of their work. CPN is a certificated course, college based and taking one year. Clinical courses are available in child and adolescent psychiatric nursing, behavioural psychotherapy, psychodynamic techniques, drug and alcohol dependency nursing, rehabilitation in residential settings, and care of the violent or potentially violent individual.

Psychiatric nurses may have felt some loss of autonomy since all services were amalgamated under the direction of a district nursing officer and all education under the director of nurse education. However, there are many benefits to be gained from being gathered into a central concern, rather than being isolated on the periphery and fighting for recognition. Now psychiatric nurses join with their general colleagues, often on the same hospital site, to be included in wider perspectives, to be involved in current issues, made easier by heightened levels of communication.

Mental handicap

There is now a total commitment to moving mentally handicapped people away from an institutional environment, to integration within the community. The whole concept has changed from custodial care with basic nursing, to a programme of training that will equip the person to function in society to their maximum ability. Two important developments in the 1970s were major influences in bringing about positive improvements to this end.

Local authorities were instructed to provide personal social services for the handicapped within the community.

The Education (Handicapped Children) Act of 1970 passed responsibility for the education of handicapped children from the health authority across to the education authority, and particularly influenced those children in long-stay care. Every child in the land, regardless of mental or physical impairment, must have some form of education between the legal school ages of five and 16. In fact, for handicapped children with special needs, this provision may span from two to 19 years of age.

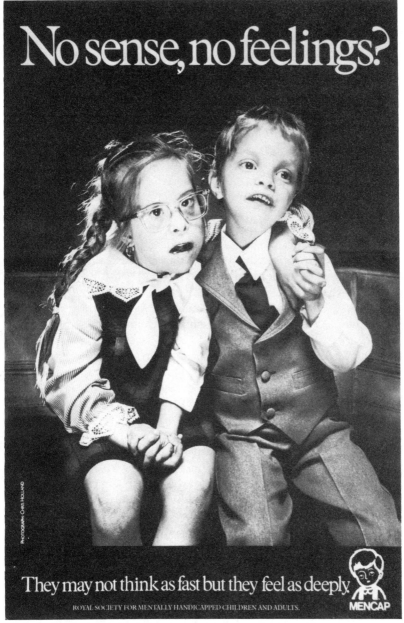

Fig. 11.5   Caring for mentally handicapped people. (Reproduced by courtesy of MENCAP.)

Children are transported from home or hospital to special schools in each area, staffed by specialist teachers, nurses, psychologists, physiotherapists and care assistants.

To the mildly handicapped (formerly known as educationally subnormal or ESN) their education concentrates to a level which their abilities will allow. It is heavily biased towards the self-care and social skills which will aid their competence in the wider community, such as reading, writing, handling money, managing in shops and public transport, using the telephone, cooking and home economics. A wide range of activities may include swimming, horseriding, horticultural therapy, as well as use of equipment borrowed from the National Toy Library Scheme.

For the profoundly handicapped, who invariably have some degree of physical handicap superimposed, the school day involves maximising their physical abilities and developing simple social skills.

All of the children benefit from the enriched and stimulating environment that the school provides. The 1981 Education Act makes provision for children with special educational needs and encourages the integration of mentally handicapped children with their peers from ordinary schools, wherever possible.

No grading system, such as IQ level, is used as a measure of mental ability in educational terms. Where there are stringent categories with cut-off points, this can limit the opportunity for development of certain skills, interests or aptitudes that the child might possess, in areas like music, art or sport.

The former terms of 'mental subnormality', 'retardation' and 'deficiency', which had acquired a derogatory stigma, have been superseded by mental 'handicap'. Gone also are references to 'high-grade' and 'low-grade' degrees of incapacity, and the use of 'profound' handicap is preferable to the term 'severe' handicap.

From the birth of a handicapped child, the parents are given positive encouragement, advised about specialist help and made aware of the many practical and financial facilities available to the family.

It is acknowledged that a normal loving home life is the best environment for any child and is equally, if not more, important for the handicapped child. Yet it is also recognised that acceptance of such a special child is a lifelong commitment, which creates an extra burden of physical and emotional responsibility on all members of the family.

Comprehensive support, advice and counselling is delivered by a community based, multidisciplinary team, who are able to assess the progress of the child and the needs of the family. The *community mental handicap team* (CMHT) will comprise a community mental handicap nurse, a social worker with special interest and possibly a psychologist, all under the overall direction of a consultant psychiatrist specialising in mental handicap. Any member of the team may draw upon the combined resources available through the services of the hospital authority or local authority.

The team is a vital contact point for families and also for other professionals who need to find out about facilities for the mentally handicapped in the borough. A register of mentally handicapped people is compiled and maintained, in order to plan services for the future.

Throughout the life of the child, it is a partnership in care between the parents and the professionals, providing opportunity for a close nurse/client relationship to be formed. Each find they are continually learning from one another, for the ultimate benefit of handicapped people as a whole.

A *family relief system* is an invaluable facility for parents who can manage to care for their child at home. They are secure in the knowledge that relief by means of temporary accommodation with professional care is available for their child in times of crisis. This may be required if the mother is ill or has another baby, if a sibling has to go to hospital or if the handicapped child himself is ill.

It is also important that parents are able to take their other children for a holiday or can get a break away by themselves, so that annual periods of residential care may be booked in advance. That precious two weeks of respite can make all the difference, it can be the crucial factor that allows a family to continue caring for the handicapped member for the remainder of the year.

If, for any reason, parents are unable to look after their child, then either a foster/adoption arrangement is secured or residential accommodation arranged. Rarely these days do children get admitted to the old-style handicap institution. Where possible they reside in a small family unit, either sited in the community or within a hospital, staffed by nurses and care assistants.

The adult mentally handicapped person beyond school-leaving age, attends an adult training centre. Here they undertake various types of employment and vocational training, suitable to their capabilities. Although it would be ideal for some handicapped people to work out in the general community, it is often difficult to find appropriate employment on the open market.

Adults transfer to adult residential accommodation, with varied types of supervision, depending upon their level of handicap and degree of social independence. This could be as warden-assisted accommodation, group home or flatlet or lodging house. In addition, recreation and leisure pursuits, holidays and church attendance needs to be offered and organised, to enrich the life of the handicapped person living in the community.

It must be remembered that a considerable number of older handicapped people have only ever known the institution where they have spent the whole of their lives. It would be difficult, and in many cases cruel, to expose them to the insecurity of the alien competitive world outside, for which they have not been prepared. The large mental hospitals are limiting admissions now but, for existing patients, provide a community setting within the grounds, arranged as small homely units for accommodation and work.

Those multiply handicapped people with profound disabilities and a high level of dependence may eventually require long-term residential care. For parents who have devoted their lives to caring for their handicapped child, their greatest concern is for the child's future prospects when the parents become infirm or die. Various trustee schemes are available to ensure the continued welfare and safeguarding of interests for the mentally handicapped person who is left alone.

Mencap

With the improved and promising outlook for mentally handicapped people, the sustained contributions of Mencap to bring about this happy situation cannot be overstated.

Modern policy is aiming towards the realisation of a dream for the Royal Society for Mentally Handicapped Children and Adults (Mencap), who have championed the cause for mentally handicapped people over many years. The embryo of the present association was formed in 1946 by a nucleus of enthusiastic, farsighted parents, who were convinced that families would be willing to care for their handicapped children, providing they were given adequate support and practical help. This was at a time when children were 'put away' in 'defective colonies', labelled as 'idiots, imbeciles or feeble-minded'.

Mencap has been committed to securing provisions for mentally handicapped people, commensurate to their needs. Another important aim has been to increase public and professional awareness of the problems faced by mentally handicapped people and their families. It is obviously necessary to create a sympathetic climate of public opinion as a prerequisite for their acceptance in the community (see Fig. 11.5).

Training

Until recently, nurses were the dominant professionals in mental handicap care, having the virtual monopoly within the bleak institutions. With staff shortage, overcrowding, limited funds and little outside interest, it was not without reason called a 'Cinderella service', where nurses struggled to do the best they could.

Then along came specialist personnel with active methods of treatment, never previously thought possible with the handicapped patients. This coincided with a wave of moral concern which swept through the nation, keen to do justice to its less fortunate members and their relatives.

The role of the nurse has had to be radically modified to keep pace with changing philosophies of care for the mentally handicapped. The transitions have been dramatic over recent years and promise to continue, as the move from institution to community accelerates.

Nurses need to be trained so they may actively participate in therapeutic regimes, such as behaviour modification, token economy therapy and social skills education. They must be fully conversant with the full spectrum of amenities available to their clients, in the form of education, recreation, occupation and vocational training. Learners must be placed within these departments to work alongside trained staff who can impart their specialist knowledge about their discipline.

A period of experience in nursing the physically ill is included in the training, as basic nursing skills can figure, to a lesser or greater extent, in the total care of the handicapped person.

In general, the syllabus has turned away from the clinical model of care and now has a social orientation. The nursing process works very well in this field of nursing, where there is a plan of individualised care.

In a community module, learners are introduced to concepts of care for the mentally handicapped in the community by working with the community team. Community mental handicap nursing (CMHN) has evolved as a specialty within this care area, for which a post-basic clinical course of training is available.

Basic training for registration (RNMH) is three years and for enrolment (ENMH) it is two years, with reductions for post-basic entrants. Nurses training for other parts of the register are also introduced to care of the handicapped, to develop all-round professional awareness.

The function of the nurse in mental handicap was seriously threatened by the notorious Jay report in 1979. In evaluating the care and service for mentally handicapped people, the report suggested that provision should be the responsibility of the social services, with training of a 'qualified care worker' to be undertaken by the Central Council for Education and Training of Social Workers (CCETSW).

This recommendation caused a major uproar in the profession, as nurses vehemently defended their position. They insisted on retaining their input and for responsibility for training to be retained by the statutory nursing body.

It is obvious that mental handicap nursing will never again be the same. But progress along positive lines of education and training can only be for the good of handicapped people.

Physical disability

For the person with a physical disability, the aim is to provide a framework of counselling, advice and practical help that will maximise his capabilities to reduce the handicap, and enable him to lead his life as independently as possible. The ultimate objective is to encourage the disabled person to function well, within the confines of his handicap, by giving a backdrop of support that will 'help him to help himself'.

The person may require assistance with any of the activities of daily living, with particular emphasis on mobility, communication, self-care and continence. A service for the physically disabled is delivered both in hospital and the community, combining the multiple expertise from a team comprising doctor, nurse, physiotherapist, occupational therapist and social worker. For patients progressing back home after a period in hospital, a home visit may be made to assess the person's particular needs within their own accommodation and to see how they manage.

Help is given across the whole spectrum of possible needs, including financial support, individualised transport and the arrangement of suitable work and holidays commensurate with their special requirements. Through the specialist skills of a domiciliary occupational therapist working with the local authority team (sometimes called a disabled living adviser) the client can be functionally assessed at home within the context of his own environment and help given toward solving problems, including self-help. A variety of gadgets and appliances may be supplied, although the help available is subject to local variation between authorities. Specialised equipment, such as hoists, ramps, cooking implements and bathroom accessories are purchased or loaned. Adaptations to houses are discussed and organised, for example providing a downstairs WC, installing a lift, widening doorways or making alterations to the kitchen or bathroom.

Physical disability may strike at any age group, manifesting a variety of handicaps. Babies may be born handicapped through cerebral palsy, spina bifida or through infection while in the uterus. The whole family needs physical, emotional and financial support to enable them to care for their special child. Early assessment of disability may involve a nurse in the primary health care team, in a community paediatric liaison service, or in special services for the handicapped.

Handicap in children

The Education Act of 1981 makes provision for children requiring special educational treatment. Rather than the old method of classifying children into fixed categories of disability of mind or body, they are assessed by their special educational needs, identified as a variety of learning difficulties and given the appropriate teaching.

Whenever practical, physically handicapped children attend an ordinary school, mixing with the mainstream pupils, and allowing them to participate in whichever general school activities they can.

There are obvious logistic difficulties to overcome before integration can be completely achieved but the idea of 'normalising' the handicapped has taken root. A high ratio of specialist staff is required, including a school nurse, physiotherapist, speech therapist and care assistants, to augment the normal teaching staff. Extensive transport arrangements are needed within the borough to get children to their school. Older buildings need to be altered to accommodate wheelchairs by adding ramps, rails, widening doors and the access to toilets.

Integration has a double-edged benefit. The disabled child is part of the general society, instead of being set apart and used only to meeting other handicapped children. He can make use of opportunities from the full range of activities offered at a normal school, is able to develop individual talents and guided into a rich and purposeful life.

Able-bodied children learn to mix freely with their handicapped colleagues, accepting that disability as one aspect of life, rather than perpetuating the stigmatised view that anyone who is different is a freak. The society ultimately benefits from a greater tolerance and understanding of handicap, starting with the next generation of adults who, as children, have been used to working side by side with friends who need special consideration.

Handicap in adults

Disability occurring in someone who has previously been fit and active presents a wider set of problems than for a child who has never known any different.

Considerable emotional and physical adjustment is required to accept the prospect of a change in lifestyle imposed by sudden blindness, deafness or paralysis following spinal injury. A similar daunting outlook accompanies the slowly developing incapacity resulting from such conditions as multiple sclerosis, rheumatoid arthritis or Parkinson's disease.

The elderly, perhaps already undermined by some infirmities of old age, may have to struggle with worsening arthritis or cope following a stroke or amputation.

In adults, the positive emphasis lies in rehabilitation to salvage remaining capabilities, combined with adaptation to a different pattern of life, accepting and overcoming the problems, as opposed to a gradual decline into depression, despair and dependence.

That grim word 'invalid', so popular for soldiers no longer fit for active service, has rightly fallen into disuse. 'Invalid' means in-valid, without validity, of no use, having no effect, null and void. None of these have a place in the modern philosophy which instils a positive outlook for the disabled person and makes every effort to include them in the full array of social activities.

It is, of course, vital that members of the person's family, as well as the community at large, recognise the varying needs of the disabled and their potential, and make allowances to integrate them smoothly into day-to-day affairs.

The legislation of 1970, the Chronically Sick and Disabled Persons Act, has seen tremendous improvements in individual help and public facilities made available for the handicapped. Local authorities have a statutory responsibility to ensure that all public premises and new public buildings are equipped for the disabled, by means of access to and within the building, and special toilet and parking facilities. The wheelchair logo is now a familiar sign in general use (Figure 11.6).

Organisations for the disabled

Other aspects of healthy living must not be denied to the physically handicapped, whose needs are the same as their able-bodied peers.

Sexual and Personal Relationships of the Disabled (SPOD) is a voluntary association concerned with the sexual aspect of life for all handicapped people.

The Physically Handicapped and Able-Bodied organisation (PHAB) arranges activities for young people, including holidays and outings, where the disabled and able-bodied youngsters share in the fun and help one another.

Sporting activities and swimming feature as part of any rehabilitation programme. Initiated from the spinal injuries centre at Stoke Mandeville Hospital, the Paralympics, or Wheelchair Olympics, are planned internationally for physically disabled competitors who excel in a variety of sporting events.

The Spastics Society is a renowned charity with a long history, which has been at the helm of many progressive landmarks relevant to disability, notably community integration and the prevention of handicap in the newborn.

A large number of voluntary organisations work with, and for, various groups of people with a specific disability, such as the deaf, the blind, the Multiple Sclerosis Society, Alzheimer's disease, Huntington's chorea and many, many more.

The Disabled Living Foundation (DLF) is a wonderful source of information regarding all services for the disabled. Advice is freely available from their information service about any aspect of help for those with special needs.

Nurses should be familiar with these organisations which have built up a tremendous wealth of knowledge and experience, and are therefore well placed to offer just the right kind of help and advice to people with a particular disability. Some organisations also provide sheltered employment or supervised housing.

With the availability of a wide variety of community services

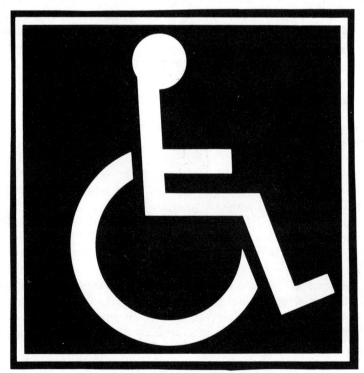

Fig. 11.6   The famous wheelchair logo.

and personnel, it is now considered the last resort for a person to be admitted for residential hospital care. However, when it does become a necessity, there are now units for the young disabled, geared to a lively, progressive rehabilitation programme for younger patients, who might otherwise have been condemned to inappropriate care on a geriatric ward.

Disabled people do not want sympathy or charity and they do not want to be a burden to the community. They do ask for the chance to take a fair crack at making a useful contribution to society, insisting that they should have the right to try by being helped to overcome their attendant obstacles.

Life with a disability is a challenge, but the disabled person wants opportunities put within his grasp—not out of all possible reach.

Holistic care and alternative therapies

So much is now understood and recognised about the inter-relation of the mind and body, that a strictly regional approach is no longer appropriate. The emotions are affected by surgery, childbirth, the menopause and the threat of serious illness, while a negative attitude can impede recovery or hasten death. Stress alters the blood pressure and anxiety affects the stomach lining and flow of gastric juices. Health is a combination of physical, emotional and social components, blending in harmony.

The holistic approach takes account of all of these factors and literally means treating 'the whole person', rather than merely attacking the most obvious symptoms. It should be the axis of all nursing care, embodied in the application of individualised patient care. Still, our medical colleagues persist in specialising to concentrate their attentions on one bodily system, as if organs function in isolation. Those in general practice are perhaps better placed to consider a holistic approach.

Certain simple general methods can be included in the umbrella title of holistic care, such as relaxation, meditation, music, art, yoga, dance, natural diet and counselling, all de-signed to enhance wellbeing and promote the balance of healthy living. Some interesting work is being done with cancer patients who are able to halt the progress of their disease by taking posi-tive health measures and use visual imagery to focus their thoughts on the tumour in order to shrink it.

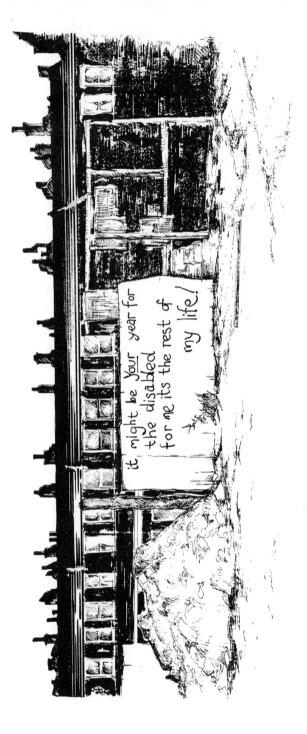

Fig. 11.7   'The rest of my life.'

Relaxation methods can be used with effect to control anxiety, and self-awareness can be a tool to alleviate depression. Orthodox medicine tends to 'take over' a patient's illness, denying him any part of controlling his destiny, and fails to take account of the self-healing properties which can be activated.

Conventional doctors have in the past been sceptical of alternative therapies and antagonistic to their use, worried about 'cranks' usurping their territory with 'quackery'. Their main face-saving excuse for this blanket opposition has always been that such methods do not lend themselves to scientific scrutiny. The happy fact that it works for some patients has never managed to vindicate that less important fact that we do not know why it works, and perhaps have no way of explaining it scientifically.

Modern medicine progressed in leaps and bounds and raised itself on a pedestal with the implication that a cure for everything would eventually be found by scientific means. For a long time that was firmly believed to be the only way, but things are gradually changing.

As chinks in the modern medical armour are demonstrated, by treatments that fail patients altogether or by treatments whose value is overshadowed by adverse side-effects, other methods are being tried. It is these people who have sought alternative help and returned singing the praises with convincing results, who have given the impetus to respect for valid alternative methods.

Many have been proven traditional treatments over many centuries before the birth of current scientific medicine and, after a period of relative obscurity, are now enjoying a new wave of interest from patients and professionals alike. One particular attraction is the 'natural' element of their healing properties, coming at a time when people are increasingly anxious about X-rays, pollutants and the ingestion of chemicals in drugs and food additives.

A respectful, although cautious, approach is developing towards this field of care. Alternative therapies do not present themselves as opponents or challengers of orthodox medicine, but offer an adjunct to existing treatments, to give a wide range of options for any patient for a particular condition. So, what used to be scathingly dismissed as 'fringe medicine' is now given the more welcoming term of 'complementary medicine'.

A new and interesting relationship is forming between conventional health workers and alternative health practitioners, both of whom are equally concerned about the charlatans who foist themselves upon an unsuspecting public with false claims.

Many therapies are organised into reputable societies, which monitor standards of training and practice and maintain a register of qualified practitioners. However, in Britain, alternative therapists do not need a state licence to practise, so there is nothing illegal in any person setting up a business offering any type of treatment. This invidious situation may have fearful consequences for patients who seek help through the small ads, rather than consulting a respected, trained practitioner.

On the other hand, if the reputable therapists and their societies are accepted as co-workers by doctors, then the patient will have at his disposal the expertise of both worlds. Currently, there is pressure to organise clinical evaluation of some of the well-established therapies, which, so far, have only been recommended on the empirical evidence of grateful patients.

Apart from homeopathy and some acupuncture, there is little provision, at present, for alternative therapies on the NHS. But some doctors are increasingly inclined to refer their patients to qualified alternative therapists and others are choosing to learn more about alternative methods and taking some training themselves. As some of the proven and established alternative treatments do gain approval, they may become more widely available for general use, especially in intractable conditions and for pain relief. The British Holistic Medical Association provides a very useful middle ground where orthodox professional and alternative therapists can find out more about the work they do and what each has to offer for the benefit of patients. It is altogether an interesting area of care that looks set to make a huge impression on total health care in the future, in both preventive and curative ways.

The following is a brief description of the principle well-established alternative therapies available.

Acupuncture

Acupuncture was used by the ancient Chinese as far back as 3000 BC but there has been a great resurgence of interest in recent years in both the East and West. The orientals use it to treat all manner of internal disorders and as an anaesthetic for performing surgery. In the West it is commonly used to alleviate chronic pain. Doctors and physiotherapists are increasingly taking the course of study which will allow them to offer acupuncture alongside their conventional methods of treatment. The principle of treatment is that fine needles are inserted at strategic points under the skin, then vibrated to alleviate pain or disease, often at a site that is anatomically unrelated to the point.

Osteopathy and chiropractic

Osteopathy and chiropractic are manipulative therapies, aimed at restoring the normal movement and function of joints, particularly in the spine. Both have a good reputation for relieving low back pain. Osteopathy is useful for sports injuries and it is not unknown to have doctors combining osteopathy with medicine and orthopaedics.

Homeopathy

Homeopathy works on the principle that physical symptoms are a manifestation of the body's fight against illness and, by giving a homeopathic remedy, it is encouraged to follow this battle through to the healed state. Remedies are often derived from herbal or mineral sources and do not suppress the body's natural response, as many modern drugs do. Several homeopathic hospitals are incorporated in the NHS and many doctors are seeking further training in this specialty. The Royal family are known to be keen advocates of homeopathic methods.

Naturopathy

Naturopathy is aimed at healthy living and the peak of fitness to obviate ill-health or reverse some disorders. It is based on good diet, alleviation of stress and reasonable exercise. Treatment would include counselling together with massage, hydrotherapy and foods which are low in fat and protein, high in fibre, often in the form of fresh raw vegetables.

Reflexology

Reflexology involves zones on the soles of the feet, which can indicate disease in some distant organ and is relieved by deep massage to the appropriate zone.

Aromatherapy

Aromatherapy employs the use of scented oils with treatment properties, usually massaged into the skin or maybe inhaled.

Therapeutic touch

Also known as laying on of hands, psychic healing or faith healing, this is based on the premise that the healer can act as a channel transferring energy to the patient, which becomes a healing agent.

Reference and refresher reading

Breakdown—Common Psychiatry for Nurses (1983). London: *Nursing Times* Publication.

Brunner L. S., Suddarth D. S. (1982). *The Lippincott Manual of Medical and Surgical Nursing* (3 vols). London: Harper and Row.

Darnbrough A., Kinrade D. (1977). *Directory for the Disabled*. Cambridge: Woodhead-Faulkner Ltd.

Eliopoulos C. (1980). *Geriatric Nursing*. London: Harper and Row.

General Nursing Council (1981). *Aspects of Sick Children's Nursing. Learning Package*. London: English National Board.

Hector W., Whitfield S. (1982). *Nursing Care for the Dying Patient and the Family*. London: Heinemann Medical Books.

Inglis B., West R. (1984). *The Alternative Health Guide*. London: Michael Joseph.

Baly M. E. with Robottom B., Clark J. and Chapple M. (1981). *A New Approach to District Nursing*. London: Heinemann Medical Books.

Intensive Care (1978). London: *Nursing Times* Publication.

Mattingley S. (1977). *Rehabilitation Today*. London: Update Publications.

Muir G., McKenzie H. (1981). *Take Care of Your Elderly Relative (A Source Book for Carers)*. London: George Allen and Unwin.

Nash W., Thruston M., Baly M. E. (1985). *Health at School: Caring for the Whole Child*. London: Heinemann Medical Books.

Owen G. M. (1983). *Health Visiting*. Eastbourne: Baillière Tindall

Psychiatry Under Review (1980). London: *Nursing Times* Publication.

Slack P. (1978). *School Nursing*. Eastbourne: Baillière Tindall.

Tierney A. J. (1983). *Nurses and the Mentally Handicapped*. Chichester: John Wiley and Sons.
Whitehead J. A. (1978). *In the Service of Old Age (The Welfare of Psycho-geriatric Patients)*. Aylesbury: HM and M Publishers.

Appendix 1

Useful addresses

UKCC—United Kingdom Central Council for Nursing, Midwifery and Health Visiting, 23 Portland Place, London W1N 3AF, tel. 01–637 7181.

ENB—English National Board for Nursing, Midwifery and Health Visiting, Victory House, 170 Tottenham Court Road, London W1P 0HA, tel. 01–388 3131.

WNB—Welsh National Board for Nursing, Midwifery and Health Visiting, 13th Floor, Pearl Assurance House, Greyfriars Road, Cardiff CF1 3RT, tel. 0222 395535.

NBS—National Board for Nursing, Midwifery and Health Visiting for Scotland, 22 Queen Street, Edinburgh EH2 1JX, tel. 031–226 7371.

NBNI—National Board for Nursing, Midwifery and Health Visiting for Northern Ireland, RAC House, 79 Chichester Street, Belfast BT1 4JE, tel. 0232–238152.

RCN—Royal College of Nursing, 20 Cavendish Square, London W1M 0AB, tel. 01–409 3333.

RCM—Royal College of Midwives, 15 Mansfield Street, London W1M 0BE, tel. 01–580 6523.

HVA—Health Visitors Association, 36 Eccleston Square, London SW1V 1PF, tel. 01–834 9523.

University of London, Department of Extra-Mural Studies, 26 Russell Square, London WC1B 5DQ, tel. 01–636 8000.

Open University PO Box 48, Milton Keynes MK7 6AB, tel. 0908–74066.

Continuing Nurse Education, Central Manchester College, Openshaw Centre, Whitworth Street, Manchester M11 2WH, tel. 061–223 8282.

Continuing Education for Nurses, Distance Learning Centre, Polytechnic of the South Bank, Manor House, 58 Clapham Common North Side, London SW4 9RZ, tel. 01–228 2015/6.

General information about careers and courses in nursing can be obtained by writing and enclosing an SAE to:

ENB Careers Advisory Centre, 26 Margaret Street, London W1N 7LB.

Scottish Health Service Centre, Crewe Road South, Edinburgh EH4 2LF.

Nurse Recruitment Officer, NI National Board, 123–137 York Street, Belfast BT15 1JB.

Appendix 2

List of Courses in Post-basic Clinical Studies of the ENB and WNB (correct as of August 1985; further details may be obtained from the respective Boards)

Long Courses Leading to the Award of a Certificate in Clinical Studies

Course Number	Nursing Subject	Eligible Candidates	Length of Course in Weeks (exclusive of holidays)
100	General Intensive Care	RGN RSCN	24 – 27
115	General Intensive Care	EN(G)	24 – 27
124	Coronary Care	RGN	17 – 19
130	Coronary Care	EN(G)	17 – 19
134	Renal and Urology	RGN	40 – 43
136	Renal	RGN	24 – 27
138	Urology	RGN	24 – 27
140	Renal and Urology	EN(G)	40 – 43
143	Renal	EN(G)	24 – 27
145	Urology	EN(G)	24 – 27
148	Neuromedical and Neurosurgery	RGN	24 – 27
153	Neuromedical and Neurosurgery	EN(G)	24 – 27
158	Paediatric Medical and Surgical Cardiothoracic	RGN RSCN	46 – 49
160	Paediatric Medical and Surgical Cardiothoracic	RSCN	36 – 39
162	Cardiothoracic	EN(G)	46 – 49
166	Cardiac Care	EN(G)	32 – 35
170	Thoracic Nursing	EN(G)	32 – 35
174	Paediatric Medical and Surgical Cardiothoracic	EN(G)	46 – 49
176	Operating Department Nursing	RGN RSCN	46 – 49
182	Anaesthetic Nursing	RGN	24 – 27
188	Operating Department Nursing	EN(G)	46 – 49
199	Accident and Emergency Nursing	RGN	36 – 39
211	Accident and Emergency Nursing	EN(G)	36 – 39
216	Stoma Care	RGN	8 – 9
219	Orthopaedic Nursing	RGN	45

Course Number	Nursing Subject	Eligible Candidates	Length of Course in Weeks (exclusive of holidays)
222	Orthopaedic Nursing	EN(G)	45
225	Gynaecological Nursing	RGN	24 – 27
228	Gynaecological Nursing	Any EN	24 – 27
237	Oncological Care	RGN	24 – 27
243	Oncological Care	EN(G)	24 – 27
249	Cardiothoracic Nursing	RGN	46 – 49
254	Cardiac Nursing	RGN	32 – 35
259	Thoracic Nursing	RGN	32 – 35
264	Burns and Plastic Surgery	RGN	36 – 39
268	Burns and Plastic Surgery	EN(G)	36 – 39
275	Nursing of Sexually Transmitted Diseases	RGN EN(G)	24 – 27
285	Continuing Care of Dying Patient and Family	RGN	8
298	Nursing Elderly People	RGN RMN RNMH Any EN	24 –27
329	Infection Control Nursing	RGN	12 over one year
338	Ear, Nose and Throat Nursing	RGN	24 – 27
344	Ear, Nose and Throat Nursing	EN(G)	24 – 27
350	Nursing Care of Physically Disabled	RGN	16 – 18
366	Nursing Care of Physically Disabled	EN(G)	16 – 18
371	Nursing Patients with Spinal Cord Lesions	RGN	24 – 27
377	Nursing Patients with Spinal Cord Lesions	EN(G)	24 – 27
382	Rheumatic Diseases Nursing	RGN	22 – 24
388	Rheumatic Diseases Nursing	EN(G)	22 – 24
393	Dermatological Nursing	RGN	24 – 27
397	Dermatological Nursing	EN(G)	24 – 27
405	Special and Intensive Care of Newborn	RGN RM RSCN	26

Course Number	Nursing Subject	Eligible Candidates	Length of Course in Weeks (exclusive of holidays)
409	Special and Intensive Care of Newborn	EN(G)	26
426	Paediatric Nursing	Any EN	42 – 45
501	Infectious Diseases Nursing	RGN	20 – 22
505	Infectious Diseases Nursing	EN(G)	20 – 22
603	Child and Adolescent Psychiatric Nursing	Any RN	46 – 49
612	Drug and Alcohol Dependency Nursing	Any RN	32 – 35
616	Drug Dependency Nursing	Any RN	20 – 22
620	Alcohol Dependency Nursing	Any RN	20 – 22
650	Adult Behavioural Psychotherapy	RMN	68 – 72
655	Rehabilitation in Residential Settings	RMN	36 – 39
660	Psychodynamic Techniques	RMN	52 – 55
705	Behaviour Modification in Mental Handicap	RNMH (Maybe other RNs)	32 – 35
805	Care of Mentally Handicapped in Community	RNMH	36 – 39
810/811	Care of Mentally Ill in Community	RMN	36 – 39

Short Courses Leading to the Award of a Statement of Competence or Statement of Attendance in Clinical Studies

Course Number	Nursing Subject	Eligible Candidates	Length of Course in Days
900	Family Planning Nursing	RM Any RN	Sessions over 14 weeks
904	Short Course of Intensive Care of Newborn	RM Any RN	15 days
906	Gastrointestinal Endoscopy	RGN EN(G)	10 – 12 days

Course Number	Nursing Subject	Eligible Candidates	Length of Course in Days
910	Principles of Infection Control	RGN	10 – 15 days
913	Care and Rehabilitation of Physically Disabled	RGN RM RSCN RMN RNMH Any EN	20 days
918	Principles of Intensive Care	Any EN	15 days
920	Principles of Intensive Care	RGN RSCN	10 days
923	Developments in Nursing Care	RGN RSCN	30 days
925	Principles of Operating Department Nursing	RGN RSCN EN(G)	10–15 days
928	Diabetic Nursing	RGN RMN RNMH RM	20 days
930	Care of Dying Patient & Family	Any RN Any EN RM	20–30 days
932	Sexually Transmitted Diseases Nursing	RGN EN(G)	5 days
933	Developments in Nursing	EN(G)	20 days
935	Advances in Mental Handicap Nursing	EM(MH)	20–30 days
936	Developments in Mental Handicap Nursing	RNMH	20–30 days
937	Behaviour Modification in Mental Handicap	Any RN Any EN	30 days
941	Nursing Elderly People	RGN RMN RNMH Any EN	22 days
945	Rehabilitation of the Mentally Ill	RMN EN(M)	20–30 days
950	Psychiatric Aspects of General Nursing	RGN RSCN RM EN(G)	20–30 days
953	Developments in Psychiatric Nursing	RMN	30 days
955	Care of Violent or Potentially Violent Person	Any RN Any EN RM	15–20 days
958	Care of Mentally Handicapped Children in Residential Settings	Any RN or EN	15 days

Course Number	Nursing Subject	Eligible Candidates	Length of Course in Days
960	Nursing Within a Secure Environment	RMN RNMH	20–30 days
963	Nursing Response to Problem Drinker	Any RN or EN RM	4–6 weeks
962	Foundation Course in Child Development	Any RN or EN	15–20 days
972	Care of Children with Multiple Handicaps	Any RN or EN	5–6 weeks
975	Care of Disturbed Children & Adolescents	Any RN or EN	25–30 days
978	Promotion of Continence & Management of Incontinence	Any RN, EN or RM	10 days
980	Principles of Stoma Care	Any RN, EN or RM	8 days
983	Care of Patients with Rheumatic Disease	RGN RSCN EN(G)	20 days
985	Principles of Psychosexual Counselling	Any RN or EN or RM	20–30 days
989	Principles of Community Psychiatric Nursing	EN (M or MH)	20–30 days
992	Community Psychiatric Nursing	RMN RNMH	20 days
995	Understanding and Application of Research	Any RN or RM	30–35 days

I wish you well.
Good luck with your plans
to return to nursing

Index